Early praise for *Living Abled and Healthy*...

"*Living Abled and Healthy* is an excellent resource for anyone facing, or helping others face, the challenge of recovering as fully as possible from an injury or illness. Well-written and comprehensive for a general audience, particularly individuals who have been injured, it addresses a real need.
 —BRIAN GOODYEAR, PHD (AUTHOR OF *THE RELENTLESS PURSUIT OF MEDIOCRITY*)

"*Living Abled and Healthy* puts forth an important message everyone needs to hear—our disability system often inadvertently creates disability rather than curing what should be temporary injuries. *Living Abled...* explains the dynamics of the disability system. This should be required reading for every medical student, insurance adjuster, lawyer, vocational rehabilitation counselor, and hearings officer!
 "As an occupational medicine physician I treated workers' compensation injuries for many years. I came to understand the incentives pulling injured workers from acute injury to permanent disability. *Living Abled...* spells out how this may evolve despite the best of intentions of both the injured worker and the treating specialists. If this book prevents even one injured worker from becoming permanently disabled, it will be worth the cost of the book a thousand times over."
 —CHUCK KELLEY, MD, MPH, MBA (CHAIRMAN, OUTRIGGER ENTERPRISES, INC.)

"This book is a bible for anyone who really wants to be well."
 —AVERYL WALLIS (HEALTHCARE CONSUMER)

"*Living Abled and Healthy* is a comprehensive and helpful book aimed at those mired in the complex world of workers' compensation—those who feel overwhelmed, frustrated, angry, and afraid. By explaining how the system works and doesn't work, how our bodies and minds function, and giving practical advice, *Living Abled...* offers hope and provides readers useful tools for getting their lives back. Written with a deep knowledge of the compensation system, work injuries, and the latest in mind-body science, the authors point a way out of the tunnel."
    —MARCOS IGLESIAS, MD, MMM (WORKERS' COMPENSATION AND
        OCCUPATIONAL MEDICINE MEDICAL DIRECTOR, MIDWEST EMPLOYERS
        CASUALTY COMPANY)

"*Living Abled and Healthy* is a wonderful and unprecedented user guide tackling the enormous complexity of dealing with one's injury and potential disability while facing the myriad variables of our various disability systems. It addresses the delicate human factors and motivators of various system players in refreshing candor, consistent with the authors' ultimate goal of empowering all patients to take control of their situations and avoid becoming needlessly disabled. Everyone will learn from this enormous effort; it should become mandatory reading for those working within disability systems and those patients entering the minefield that these very systems can become!"
    —BOB STEGGERT (RETIRED VICE PRESIDENT, CASUALTY CLAIMS,
        MARRIOTT INTERNATIONAL)

"The biggest takeaway... is this: Every new day offers us the chance to recreate ourselves, to stay open to the moment. When we are not who we were, we can become who we will be... We can learn from others who fully embrace life despite what some might see as impossible barriers."
  —TARA WHITE, RN (AMERICAN CHRONIC PAIN ASSOCIATION)

"Injury, illness, and disability... can be maddeningly complex and frustrating... *Living Abled and Healthy* will help anyone negotiate this labyrinth and emerge a more complete and whole person."
  —LARRY DOSSEY, MD (AUTHOR OF *REINVENTING MEDICINE* AND
    ONE MIND)

"Everyone is familiar with the concept of work-life balance. Yet, in our healthcare system, the 'work' part is dramatically underweighted. Every day, thousands of physician-patient encounters end without a single consideration of the effects of the injury or illness on employment and productivity. The results of this negligence are tragic. The authors boldly call out the perverse incentives, bureaucracy, and misinformation that plague 'disability.' They urgently challenge providers and patients to reform their thinking about the whole person—fully incorporating the reality that one's occupation is fundamental to physical and emotional health."
  —JON SEYMOUR, MD (FORMER PRESIDENT, GUIDELINES, REED GROUP)

"Thought provoking and controversial and leaves no sacred cow unscathed."
    —STEVEN BABITSKY, JD (PRESIDENT, SEAK, INC.)

"*Living Abled and Healthy* is the first book I have read that speaks openly and honestly about the importance of nutrition, the value of attitude, the concepts and perception of pain, and the tolerance and time required for physical-mental-emotional healing.
    "Recognizing the importance of protein, the importance of overall attitude, and the need to focus on a positive future, of not settling for a diagnosis that is less than tolerable, makes *Living Abled...* a guidance manual for all within the illness and injury community."
    —ROSEMARY MCKENZIE-FERGUSON (WORK INJURED RESOURCE
        CONNECTION INC., AUSTRALIA)

"*Living Abled and Healthy* is about transforming lives for the better. Beyond the personal benefit of taking responsibility for our individual health and lifestyle choices, *Living Abled...* reminds us of our responsibility to care for one another.
    "From homes to physician offices, work cubicles to boardrooms, *Living Abled...* should be required reading by everyone involved in our healthcare-delivery system."
    —BILL GILMOUR (PRESIDENT, BIOMOTION OF AMERICA)

Living Abled & Healthy

Your Guide to Injury & Illness Recovery

Living
Abled & Healthy

Your Guide to
Injury & Illness
Recovery

Christopher R. Brigham, MD

with Henry Bennett

Healthy Living Publishing

Honolulu

Inquiries should be addressed to:
Healthy Living Publishing, LLC
P.O. Box 1500
Kailua, Hawai'i 96734
publisher@healthylivingpublishing.com

Printed on acid-free paper ∞
First Edition
ISBN-13: 978-0-9634454-2-1
ISBN-10: 0-9634454-2-1
Printed in the United States of America
21 20 19 18 17 16 15   6 5 4 3 2 1

Notice: The content is not intended to be a substitute for professional medical advice,
diagnosis, or treatment nor for legal or other advice. Always seek medical advice from
a qualified medical professional. Please do not disregard, avoid, or delay obtaining
medical or health-related advice from your healthcare professional or advice about
other issues from other professionals because of anything you may read in *Living
Abled and Healthy*. Please consult your doctor or other healthcare professional before
beginning or changing any health or fitness program.

Neither the authors, the publisher, nor its dealers or distributors shall be liable to the
purchaser or any other person or entity with respect to any liability, loss, or damage
caused or alleged to be caused directly or indirectly by *Living Abled and Healthy* or
the content presented herein.

The content of sections supplied by additional contributors reflects the opinions of
the contributors.

Living Abled and Healthy is dedicated to those who,

despite injury or illness,

take control and experience joyful, productive lives.

Contents

Preface

During our lives we will deal with injury or illness and we will recover—or we may not. There is a significant chance we or someone we care about will become disabled. For over three decades, as a clinician and as a researcher focusing on health and disability issues, I have pondered:

- What defines disability and how may it be prevented?
- Why do people with similar problems, even when they receive the same care, sometimes have dramatically different outcomes?
- How do compensation systems, healthcare professionals, and our own actions contribute to our health or disability?
- How are we best able to experience joyful and productive lives?

I have been motivated by people who, despite catastrophic injuries or illnesses, live inspirational lives. I have been saddened by others who have been trapped in a needless belief of being disabled. I have been impressed by skillful, caring doctors. I have been appalled by others who misuse trusting individuals for personal financial gain.

I have been blessed with the experience of evaluating and managing several thousands of patients and working with countless skilled colleagues in dealing with the problems of these patients. I have researched and written hundreds of professional publications and learned there are no easy answers.

We need to shift from our current focus on disability to one targeting ability. We cannot passively wait for such a change when each of us may act to improve our health and ability.

C.R.B

Introduction

My back hurts. Is it from work or from being rear-ended two weeks ago? Did it just happen? What am I going to do? Do I need to go see someone? Should I rest up or should I just try to ignore the pain and push through? Do I need x-rays? Should I find a lawyer? Is it going to get better or last forever? I'm confused and scared. Where can I get answers I can trust?

We all hate being hurt or sick. It gets worse if, at the same time, we have to deal with challenging medical, legal, insurance, disability, and financial issues. Sometimes the questions, people, and systems we face make our lives really difficult.

Life should not have to be this way. But, today, since it is, *Living Abled and Healthy* is a guide for our taking charge during injury or illness rather than allowing others to take charge of us. Maneuvering through medical and legal systems may not be easy and the answers are not always clear. Using what is shared here will help us in living healthier and more productive lives.

"Disabled" is distinguished from "abled." "Disabled" is defined as "activity limitations and/or participation restrictions in an individual with a health condition, disorder, or disease." "Abled" is a less commonly seen word. "Abled" is defined as "having a full range of physical or mental abilities; not disabled." Here the strongest use of "abled" is to define us as capable of successfully living healthy and productive lives whether or *not* we still have our "full range" of abilities.

Throughout *Living Abled and Healthy* we will use the term "we" in

1

the inclusive sense. We believe that "we"—you and I and I and everyone else—all face the same issues.

❦ ❦ ❦

Injury, illness, and aging are all part of living. For our best chance at happy and healthy lives we need to understand our bodies.

Modern "Western" medicine has been based on "biomedical" models focusing on biological/mechanical approaches to injury and illness. To better understand injury, illness, and disability, we embrace a "biopsychosocial" approach including biological, psychological, and social elements. Physical illnesses we face affect all of who we are—including our minds and spirits. Our mind-body connections are surprisingly strong. If we believe something is helping us we will likely feel better. If we believe something is hurting us we will likely feel worse.

- Have we ever faced injury or illness and been unsure of what to do?
- Have we ever questioned whether medical care we received or did not receive represented the best decisions?
- Have we ever wondered if we might have more actively shared in decision-making along with our healthcare providers?
- Have we ever wondered what actually caused our problems and what we could be doing to keep them from affecting us for so long—maybe forever?
- Have we ever questioned whether we should continue working or apply for disability compensation?
- Have we ever wondered whether our lawyers were focused on helping us or on helping themselves?
- Have we ever been overwhelmed by the sheer complexity of the systems surrounding our healthcare?
- Have we ever wondered how best to deal with our emotions when we face losses and frustrations?

At one time or another pretty much all of us have.

❦ ❦ ❦

Our medical, legal, and disability "systems" are not always healthy. Instead of an organized whole, they operate as fragmented parts.

Sometimes organizations and individuals appear more focused on what benefits them than on what benefits us. Most of the people we meet act from their hearts—some don't. Systems, healthcare professionals, and procedures intended to help us can sometimes hurt us.

Profit incentives affect many stakeholders and sometimes drive actions that are not in our best interests. Those of us in the United States not enrolled in health maintenance organizations (HMOs) generally pay our doctors on a "fee for services" basis for doing things. The emphasis is on doctors finding and fixing our injury or illness, rather than helping us stay healthy. Involving lawyers in our injury or illness recovery is sometimes necessary. However, the U.S. legal system (as well as many others) is designed so that plaintiff's lawyers, those representing us, typically make more money if we become identified as seriously injured, ill, or disabled.

Americans live shorter and less healthy lives than residents of other developed nations—while paying more. This must be recognized as a national crisis and addressed through political and economic reform and through changes in our behaviors and expectations. Workers' compensation and other insurance programs rarely compensate us for the full personal effects of our injuries—and were never intended to do so.

Doctors, lawyers, and employers/insurers are the three main players in our medical care, each with their own perspectives and goals. We can compare their efforts to the "balance of power" concept expressed in the United States Constitution. A functional system needs checks and balances. Doctors, lawyers, and employers/insurers are heavily influenced by often-competing (but sometimes shared) financial incentives. We are caught in the middle.

Our lives will be affected by the individuals we meet who are or who represent these players. Some individuals will be more honest and caring than others.

This does not mean the medical, legal, and employment professionals we interact with are bad people. Often it just means they are doing what they were taught to do. They are simply responding to the systems in which they work and the ways in which they are rewarded.

We are blessed with many excellent doctors and other healthcare professionals. Some, however, may not always focus on our "health"—

particularly on our health as viewed with a "whole person" perspective. Some doctors may, instead, focus on ordering tests, prescribing medications, and providing treatments. Sometimes they focus on tests and treatments because they have good reasons to fear possible legal repercussions from *not* doing these things. Sometimes doctors behave this way because it is what *we* have asked for—or even demanded.

Many of our health problems may be prevented or at least improved through healthy lifestyle choices involving diet, exercise, not smoking, not using alcohol and/or other drugs to excess, and basically just not abusing our bodies. Improving our health may not necessarily require medical treatments—we may simply need to make the right lifestyle choices and stick with them.

Think about our cars. We maintain cars so they don't break down and make us spend even more money having them fixed.

We will sometimes face injuries or congenital or hereditary illnesses or other conditions with no known explanations and which cannot be associated with anything we did or we failed to do. Despite our best efforts, and those of our doctors, we may become sick and face challenging lives. This can be extremely frustrating and depressing. The best we can do is to approach life as courageously and as positively as we can, one day at a time.

❦ ❦ ❦

Living Abled and Healthy offers principles for healthy living and for recovering from injury or illness. For some of us, some of these principles may be new:

- Taking control of our life and health
- Staying positive
- Partnering with quality healthcare providers practicing evidence-based and data-driven medicine
- Approaching health problems from a "biopsychosocial" perspective
- Weighing the risks and benefits of testing and treatment
- Focusing on a healthy body, mind, and spirit
- Choosing smart lifestyles including exercise, diet, and health habits

- Weighing the risks and benefits of involving lawyers
- Cooperating with other healthcare participants and avoiding unnecessary conflict
- Continuing with our jobs, if at all possible

If we make use of the principles offered, the information shared, and the resources provided in *Living Abled and Healthy* and at www. livingabled.com, we may be better able to control our health decisions and live happier lives.

Health and Work

I hurt. I feel sick. What IS healthy, anyway? I don't understand my healthcare system. I just see one doctor after another—all they seem to do is to order more and more tests and write more and more prescriptions. My problems are hurting my family, particularly the kids. What should I do?

What does it really mean to be healthy? The World Health Organization (the public-health unit of the United Nations) defined health as "a state of complete physical, mental, and social well-being and not merely the absence of disease or infirmity." This is a broad definition. It recognizes that health encompasses body, mind, and spirit. It is such a broad definition that probably, by this standard, none of us could claim to be perfectly healthy. Most of us would probably agree that health is our ability to function—to do the things we want to do and need to do and interact with others and our environment.

In the United States—if we are at all honest with ourselves—we must admit we really do not have a healthcare "system." In the United States we have a largely reactionary system focusing on our injuries or illnesses rather than on our health. Fragmented components of a medical industry do not constitute a system. This is costly and inefficient. Despite this, for some practitioners working within healthcare, it may be extremely profitable.

Do most doctors really assist us in working toward that description of "complete physical, mental, and social well-being"? Some do; particularly primary care providers who take the time to address prevention. Others do not.

The way most medical care is provided does not support or reward or, in some cases, even allow doctors to work toward that description of our total health. The training we provide doctors does not, for the most part, give them the skills or allow them the time to work toward this goal. Our insurance systems typically do not pay doctors for spending the needed time with us. Our medical schools focus on injury and illness, not on promoting health.

What does influence our health? First we would have to recognize the importance of genetics—the way bodies, like snowflakes, are all different. But genetics only determines where we start. Experiences, personal health practices, and lifestyle choices greatly shape where we end up. The more we know about how to care for our bodies, and the more we practice what we know, the healthier we are likely to be.

Physical, social, and work environments all affect health. How much money we have and our social status affect our health. If we do not have adequate resources, we may not get the best possible healthcare. In the worst of situations we may not get any healthcare at all.

While we cannot yet change our genetics or some of the things that happen to us, we do make many choices affecting our health. We can choose to live a healthy lifestyle. We can eat right, stay physically fit, maintain an appropriate weight, do our best to sleep well, not smoke, and not abuse alcohol and/or other drugs. Our choices are important factors in whether or not we stay healthy.

We need to be honest with ourselves. We can make healthy choices. Or we can choose to eat junk food, not exercise, smoke, and use too much alcohol and/or other drugs. While, at the time, we may enjoy some things we know are bad for us, we need to remind ourselves that not being able to be active with loved ones and friends, being overweight, and just feeling lousy do not make for a happy life—and will usually shorten whatever life we do have.

If we truly care about the life we live, our health—our ability to function, now and long term—must guide our choices. Not all choices are easy—but we can choose.

Our Families and Communities

Most of us will not experience the challenges of injury, illness, or disability in isolation. Most of us are members of families and communities. Our interactions with our families and communities are always complex. Our experiences affect our families and communities and the reactions of our families and communities affect our experiences.

Barbara suffers from long-lasting pain throughout her body. She reports, "I feel like my life, as I knew it, was taken from me. I used to hike and swim all the time. Now I'm in constant pain and take medications and live with their side effects.

"I rarely cook—I buy fast food for my children and myself. I am irritable with my children and my husband—so none of them really want to be around me. My husband now drinks more and I see him less. Because of my pain, we are no longer intimate. I can't seem to escape."

Barbara was labeled as having chronic pain. She has become less active and more easily fatigued, more irritable, and suffers from depression. Barbara's mental and physical health is spiraling downward—and she is dragging her family down with her.

When we have health issues we change the dynamics of our interactions. Where we once may have offered support to our families and communities we may now be seeking or in need of support from them. Our new roles will likely change how we are perceived. If we are less able to function, others may have to assume the tasks we once performed, increasing their burdens. This may result in resentment or force others to assume new roles. Sometimes new roles will leave individuals feeling more empowered and valued; other times a new role may leave someone feeling less empowered and less valued.

Our families and communities affect how we respond to injury or illness or possible disability. If we are lucky, they encourage us and serve as our advocates. Not all of us will be lucky. Overly sympathetic family and community members may reinforce our perceptions of injury or illness. Some, consciously or unconsciously, will use our problems to increase their empowerment while decreasing ours. Family and community members may help create or reinforce our sense of being a victim.

The best of our family and community members will offer us "tough love"—limited sympathy coupled with high expectations for our own efforts. The best advice we may get will be to stay active and always focus on improving our situation. Responses we may see as harsh may help drive us to greater efforts and actually benefit us.

When we are the family or community member facing the injury or illness or possible disability of someone for whom we care, we want to be positive and encouraging. We should reinforce the efforts of those we care about to promote function, face challenges, and stay or become empowered. We need to provide to those we care about the benefits of our "tough love."

We should encourage their greatest possible activity rather than their excessive rest. We must support their healthy lifestyle choices and never encourage a focus on pain or on how bad they feel. As best as we can, we want to demonstrate healthy lifestyle choices in our own lives.

When those we care about have been physically or sexually abused or are dealing with other difficult life situations, we may encourage them to seek the assistance of qualified counselors—being careful that we never act to diminish their own independence, self-reliance, and empowerment. We can offer to help identify appropriate healthcare providers, looking for those professionals truly working to facilitate recovery. No matter what issues those we care about may be facing, we should always encourage them to be as active as possible and, if at all possible, to resume their prior activities and quickly return to their jobs.

Our Children

Our childhoods are the foundation upon which we build our lives. As children we learn from how we see others live their lives. In the best of all worlds these will be empowering examples.

Life Without Limits

In 1982 in Brisbane, Australia, Nick Vujicic was born without arms or legs. Missing limbs have not stopped him from living what he describes as a "ridiculously good life." Vujicic's childhood was challenging. He faced bullying, self-esteem issues, and difficulties with depression and loneliness.

But from the beginning, his parents always encouraged him to maximize his potential. They found solutions so that he could get along by himself. At seventeen Vujicic started his own non-profit organization, "Life Without Limbs." He presents motivational speeches worldwide on life lived with physical limitations. He speaks of hope and of finding meaning in life. His family, friends, and others whose lives he has touched encouraged him to document his life's story in Life Without Limits *and other publications.*

Vujicic attributes his success to his religious faith and his belief in having a purpose. Married and a father, he has a passion for life and has embraced life well beyond his apparent limitations. He now inspires others.

Not all of us will have lived in the best of all worlds. As children we may have watched parents or other relatives demean each other, us, or others. Comments such as "you're not smart enough," "you're stupid," or "you're bad" may have damaged our ability to develop empowered, independent, and self-reliant problem-solving skills.

If we become parents, our children will learn from us. If we had a positive childhood, our children will likely reap the benefits of the positive life experiences we will emulate with little effort. They will see and learn from our empowered, independent, and self-reliant responses as we deal with life's challenges. They benefit when we model healthy lifestyles including diet, exercise, and other sensible choices. Living the best lives we can will help teach our children to live the best lives they can.

If we faced abusive, demeaning, or unpleasant childhoods, we must fully recognize the histories we carry and consciously work at fighting ingrained negative behaviors to offer our children a better future. We need to consciously and consistently work to provide our children with opportunities to develop empowered, independent, and self-reliant problem-solving skills. We can become the role models we needed when we were children.

Disablement may also begin early in life. Labeling at an early age with the vague and controversial labels currently assigned to more and more young children cannot fail to influence self-identity. Some of us who simply might have been "difficult" students or "problems" in earlier generations are now labeled as "school dysfunctional" or "disabled." Unnecessary labeling may lead to self-perception of disability and later overdependence on healthcare providers.

Character is made up of attitudes and behaviors we acquire over time. Consideration of others, moral values, self-responsibility, and work habits are functions of character. Parents generally play major roles in developing our characters—often more by how they live than by what they teach. Personalities are initially shaped in childhood, and early personality traits—and possibly personality disorders—may define us for the rest of our lives.

Negative parenting is well-recognized to be a generational problem often passed down within families. But it does not need to be. Early emotional relationships directly affect the first years of brain growth and development. We can ensure our children will not be given the wrong tools to later pass on to their children. One generation of positive parenting—ours—can stop this cycle and begin better lives for all who follow.

A positive childhood is the most valuable gift we can pass on to our children. Our ability to live empowered, independent, and self-reliant lives begins with our childhood.

Work is—Gasp!—Good for Us

Many of us gripe about going to work. Getting up and going to our jobs may feel like a chore, something we push ourselves to do day in and day out. And it certainly is worse if we actually do not enjoy our jobs or find our jobs fulfilling. Despite this, the documented truth—and a truth most of us recognize deep inside even when we'd rather not admit it—is that our going to our jobs *is* good for us.

Work is, in general, good for our health and well-being. Even when we may not be making a lot of money, we know we are in better financial shape by working than if we were not working. Most of us recognize this quickly when we face those times we cannot work, cannot find work, or are denied work.

When we enjoy and respect our jobs, our work often helps us to establish who we are, our identities, and our status. Work may provide us a sense of community and social inclusion. Work may allow us to make a contribution to society.

But again, even when we do not really enjoy our jobs, we know that work contributes to our self-respect and supports us and lets us support our families. Even with less-than-perfect jobs we usually benefit from that shared sense of community and social inclusion.

Work provides us structure and ensures that we get at least some daily physical activity—even when our activity may be little more than getting to and from our jobs every day. Work gives us a reason—a need—to get up daily.

Surprisingly, work actually provides us one of the major therapeutic ingredients for pain relief—distraction. This is a simple reality. The more we focus on our jobs the less we focus on our discomfort.

Working decreases our likelihood of smoking and/or abusing alcohol and/or other drugs or of engaging in other risky behaviors. Working combats the greatest psychological threat for all of us experiencing chronic pain—spending too much of our time and thought focused on pain and other symptoms (sensations). Even when dealing with injury or illness, staying at work or quickly returning to work can be beneficial to our health and well-being.

Not Working is *Not* Good for Us

Our health risks from not working are largely the opposites of what we recognize as our benefits from working.

Not working places us at greater risk of poorer physical and mental health, long-standing illnesses, psychological distress, increased use of healthcare resources, and death. Those of us dealing with long-term unemployment or those who have never worked are two-to-three times more likely to have poor health than those who are working.

Work may be risky—many jobs have significant elements of actual physical danger. Reliable scientific studies have shown, however, that our health risk from not working is actually greater than it is from working even some risky jobs—such as working construction on the North Sea.

Losing—or never having generated—income can be extremely damaging to our self-respect. Our overall rate of suicide increases by six times if we do not work for a long period. Studies document that when we have no job we suffer from increased rates of heart disease, lung cancer, and respiratory infections. We also have more bodily complaints, see healthcare providers more often, take more drugs, and end up in the hospital more often when we are not working. Some of this is caused by our increased poverty when we have no jobs. Not working affects our opportunities for future employment.

Those of us who leave disability compensation and return to our jobs usually see improvements in income, socio-economic status, and health and general well-being. How much positive effect we get from re-employment may depend on the security of our jobs and on our desires, motivations, and job satisfaction.

Not working may leave us with psychological and social wounds we may pass along to our children and our children's children. Long-term feelings of a lack of worth are one of our greatest known public-health risks. Families where neither parent has recently worked face a higher likelihood of long-lasting and recurring illnesses, increased bodily complaints, and diminished well-being. In families where neither parent has a job, our children are more likely to lack jobs in the future. When parents face increased economic pressures, children may experience psychological distress or display delinquent behaviors.

Staying At and Returning To Our Jobs

When jobs are in short supply for everyone it becomes even more difficult for us to return to work following an injury or illness—particularly if we now face some form of physical limitation. When there are more potential workers than available jobs, employers are less likely to accommodate individuals with additional needs. Clearly, if we have been working and become injured or ill, we want to do everything we can to preserve our jobs.

The longer we are out of work for injury or illness the less likely we are to return to work. If we are off work for twenty days, our chance of ever returning to work is 70 percent. If we are off work for forty-five days, our chance of ever returning to work decreases to 50 percent. If we are off work for seventy days, our chance of ever returning to work drops even further to 35 percent. To reduce our risk of becoming disabled, we want to continue in our jobs, even if we might be injured or ill (as long as doing so will not actually harm us or pose a threat to others)—or return to work as quickly as we possibly can.

Many of us who have been advised we cannot work will have been given this advice because of muscle, tendon, bone, or mental-health conditions rather than because of any catastrophic or life-threatening injury or disease. Lower-back pain is the leading cause for years of work lost to disability. Often just being out of work may cause or add to our health problems. Studies reveal that many of our problems are affected by our attitudes towards jobs and family situations.

Only a small fraction of our medically *excused* days off work are medically *required*. We can generally work and be productive as long as we have no specific medical condition actually stopping us from working.

Medically *discretionary* absences occur when we or our employers do not make the extra effort we need to find a way to stay at work.

It is often difficult for doctors to say "no" when we ask if we can stay away from work. Our treating doctors are typically loyal and want to please. They are concerned about refusing to approve medical absences and our then becoming injured at work.

Many doctors may not be familiar with the scientific data on problems associated with being away from work. We need to insist that our doctors focus on functional ability. Before asking doctors to assess possible disability, *we* must make certain they understand how to assess our ability to work, the administrative systems we and they must address, and how best to communicate with both us and our employers.

Our ability to work is determined by three factors: risk, capacity, and tolerance.

Risk refers to problems we might likely encounter that may threaten our health while we perform a certain task if we have a medical condition. It must be judged scientifically on the specifics of our medical situation and the tasks we need to accomplish.

Capacity is what we are able to do. Often we may limit ourselves by believing we can do less than what we actually can. Sometimes we may overestimate our capabilities.

Tolerance refers to our ability to cope with symptoms (sensations). Discomfort does not mean we can't do something—it only means we experience a sensation.

We may limit ourselves because we fear our symptoms will get worse with activity. The best of evidence-based medicine tells us that increasing our activity often actually decreases our symptoms.

A doctor simply asking if we can return to work does not effectively determine if we can work. Doctors need to medically determine our functional ability. Doctors must take the time to understand our job requirements and assess whether or not we can meet those requirements. Employers should use this information to determine what we can do and what accommodations we may need.

If we are returning to work after an injury or illness, and our jobs are physically demanding, we may reasonably expect our employers to initially minimize the most difficult aspects of our jobs. Employers may start us back with limited times or limited tasks and increase our responsibilities as we regain our conditioning.

If injury or illness results in our being at risk for certain work activities or we lack the required capacity, our doctors and others should help us in receiving the compensation we deserve. This includes providing the information needed to qualify us for compensation on a timely basis. Life is difficult enough when we are injured or ill—and even more difficult if we are no longer receiving the money we need.

Employers must value us as human beings and be willing to work with us as employees. Some employers are better than others at valuing us and actively engaging us when we face physical and/or psychological challenges. Smart employers are open to modifying jobs and schedules to maintain people at work and encouraging early return to work. Other employers may not be so enlightened.

Smart employers value us as employees and recognize that we are the heart of their organizations. Smart employers ensure that workplaces are safe and create a culture of health and well-being. They value positive relationships between supervisors and staff. Smart employers do everything possible to help those injured or ill continue to work and accommodate our return to work.

When we have been out of work, smart employers facilitate "three way contact" involving us, them, and our doctors to achieve a shared goal of our returning to work as quickly as possible. Employers may involve case managers to assist in this process.

The benefits of promptly returning to work have been rigorously tested in extensive scientific studies. Scientists and doctors have, since ancient times, studied the relationship between work and well-being and have repeatedly confirmed these conclusions.

In the 1990s it became possible to gather and study patient data regarding the length of our time off work relative to specific medical conditions. Experts began developing insights about why certain conditions create longer work absences. The patterns identified helped healthcare providers better understand which parts of a typical absence are really needed. Strategies were devised to help us return to work as our normal healing processes increase our capacity. Publications expressing these insights are recognized as "disability duration guidelines." We will examine these guidelines further in chapter 4, "What Do We Mean?"

What Do We Do?

We recognize that our health is our responsibility. We help ourselves and others by maintaining a positive attitude about recovery. We recognize the value of our jobs and do not accept doctors telling us we cannot work unless they can offer us good evidence. We recognize that our working is generally healthy and that our not working is generally unhealthy. We tell our doctors and employers we intend to continue working but we may need accommodations—because working is better for us.

2

Taking Control of Our Health

*I was so angry about the accident. It was such a relief
to get beyond that.
My primary care doctor helped me understand that
I control my life. I can choose to focus on my health—
body, mind, and spirit.*

Managing Our Lives

We all need to take and keep control of our lives, including our health. When we have a health challenge, we need to identify our best resources and then take action. Even more important than our choice of medical treatment or possible legal guidance is our state of mind.

We need to understand that health and other challenges are simply part of life. Challenges are opportunities for growth. Growth may be painful but it is key to our lives. When we change our thinking and our beliefs we change our lives. No one else may be allowed to dictate our lives. Our moments of doubt must not be exploited by others.

Attitudes shape lives, create meaning, and define destinies. Being resilient and claiming empowerment can make all the difference. Passiveness limits our opportunities and gives to others what should be our control.

Drug advertisements we hear, read, and see every day in the United States tell us to "Ask your doctor if (Brand X) is right for you." Better questions would be "Do we really need any drugs?" and "Would better lifestyle decisions solve our problems and leave us healthier?" Lifestyle decisions may often offer greater benefits than drugs.

Healthy Minds

Deciding whether we are or are not healthy or disabled is as much about how we see ourselves as it is about our physical realities. Are we positive or negative? We need to believe in ourselves and believe in our positive futures.

It's All Attitude

Lou Darnell is a U.S. Army colonel retired from active duty who heads up a telecommunications company in Hawai'i. He has faced various health challenges, including those of prostate cancer and kidney disease. Despite being diagnosed with these diseases he faces life with vigor. At sixty-eight, wanting to maintain his mental and physical health, he continued running his business and decided to start riding a bicycle.

Darnell later had a heart attack, causing him to fall down a flight of stairs. He was knocked unconscious and suffered serious hip and shoulder injuries. During his recovery he stayed determined, combating his discomfort with ever-increasing activity.

Within two weeks Darnell was cautioned by his cardiologist about the risks of aggressive riding, but jointly they felt the risks versus the benefits were such that Darnell could return to biking. He heard about a bike ride honoring a local university student bicycle-safety advocate. At eighteen, Zachary Manago had been killed in a collision with a hit-and-run driver while biking.

Six months following Darnell's heart attack, he completed the 145 mile bike ride around the island of O'ahu, Hawai'i, in memory of Manago.

Darnell was the oldest rider in the event but he out-rode many others who were half his age.

His motto is "Know your goals and priorities and approach them with a positive attitude."

A positive attitude helps us to focus on our strengths, understand but ignore our weaknesses, and move on with our lives. While we cannot change the things that have happened, we can change our attitude. It is simply a matter of choice.

History—We all have pasts—some better, some worse. Our past is only a memory to which our present gives meaning. Today we may be dealing with the consequences of an injury or illness and we may need to redefine who we are.

Some of us have been lucky to have had nurturing families who helped us develop strong coping skills. Others of us became too accepting and expecting of being nurtured and never developed any self-reliance.

Some of us have had rough lives. Maybe we were victimized as children. We may feel that the world is out to get us—and we may end up always living as victims. Others of us have lived lives as rough or rougher but have only come away tougher than when we started.

Because our brains change throughout our lives (which we'll talk more about later) our experiences shape, but do not control, our lives.

Some of us have histories that still haunt us—traumatic mental or physical injuries or sexual abuse. Maybe we did not have a nurturing home. Maybe we have faced really bad work situations or suffered bad experiences with healthcare providers or insurers. These histories can profoundly affect our present. But histories are simply that—things that happened in the past.

There is what actually happened to us and then there is the meaning we give to our pasts. We may blame a painful condition on an injury and have strong feelings associated with the incident and, possibly, the people involved. If we focus too strongly on past events, we find ourselves trapped, unable to move forward.

The Present—Every new day offers us the chance to re-create ourselves, to stay open to the moment.

Many who have sustained catastrophic injuries, lost limbs, or suffered damaged spinal cords have chosen to live joyful and productive lives.

How do we make such choices? We recognize that we are not our history. Our situations and patterns of behavior help create our experiences. With awareness we can change our situations and behaviors. Acceptance of the past is part of making our choice.

Fear and worry hurt us. Negative thoughts trap us. Our minds tend to make real what we believe. We want to do our best to be as optimistic as we can be.

Anger is a heavy burden to carry. Whether it is anger toward others or toward ourselves, it is still a burden. Whether or not we are factually right in our beliefs about the causes of our problems, our anger is still an anchor holding us back from moving forward.

This is a particular challenge where, as with vehicle or other accidents or workplace injuries, there are insurance claims or litigation. If we focus too much on our perception of the cause of our problems, and are required to repeatedly demonstrate to others the severity of these problems and concentrate on retribution, we may do even more damage to ourselves.

"If we have to prove we are ill, we can't get well" is one way these thoughts might be expressed. While circumstances may dictate that we go through the claims or litigation processes, we want to minimize unhealthy thinking that only magnifies our problems.

If we are injured in a vehicle accident, at work, or from other circumstances, we may be entitled to certain compensation. But unless we forgive, whether it is others, ourselves, or just the situation, it will be hard for us to move forward. While we absolutely should obtain the care and compensation we deserve, we need to focus on the event as history, not give it overwhelming emotion, and forgive. We must take command of our present and look to a brighter future.

Gratitude—Multiple scientific studies have demonstrated a relationship between gratitude and increased well-being. When we are injured or ill we may find it difficult to feel or express gratitude. But not recognizing those aspects of our lives for which we should be grateful only harms us. Negativity only hurts us. We can focus on how injured or ill we are or we can focus on how we are not more injured, more ill, or dead.

Resiliency—We vary in our ability to cope with stress and adversity. Some of us bounce back quickly to our earlier levels of successful functioning. Some of us have to work harder.

We may process adversity, such as injuries or illness, to grow and become stronger. Resiliency is learned, starting with childhood. If our environment promotes well-being and teaches us how to address and avoid risk factors, we will become more resilient. If we practice coping effectively with small stresses, we become more resilient and better prepared to handle bigger stresses.

We want to develop good problem-solving skills, to recognize when and from where we should seek support. Sometimes we will find support from family, friends, or healthcare providers.

We need to recognize when external circumstances cannot be changed and develop rational goals to make the best of our realities. We should strive with self-confidence for ever-improving lives.

Stress—We all face stress. Stress is the body's response to a challenge. Our stress may be driven by both positive (job promotions or new and evolving relationships) and negative (becoming injured or ill) changes in our lives.

Sooner or later we all face the stress of some hardship or trauma. What is important is how we respond—how we develop a toughness of body, mind and spirit.

Chronic stress may harm our brain. Long-term exposures to stress hormones, such as cortisol, affect our bodies. Stress may produce physical symptoms, some of which we may attribute to injury or illness, such as headaches, muscle and spinal pains, and fatigue. When we are stressed we will likely stress those around us—especially those who care the most about us.

How do we manage stress? We can choose healthy ways to manage and reduce our stress. We can seek out calming surroundings. When possible, we can delegate some of our responsibilities to others. For many of us it helps to spend time in meditation, prayer, yoga, or other mindful practices.

One of our best treatments for stress is laughter. Play and laughter are therapeutic and even strengthen our immune systems. Learning to laugh at our lives and ourselves can be lifesaving—it offers great benefits with no risks.

Relationships—Relationships are critically important to our health. Relationships with our family and friends must be nurtured. Their support for and loyalty to us strengthens us.

Goals—We may only wander through our lives unless we define and work toward goals. Goals often include emotional, financial, intellectual, physical, social, spiritual, or work success. We may find greater success when we set times and measures for our goals.

For our recovery from injury or illness, we want to identify specific goals and the steps we will take to achieve them. The more clearly we define our goals the greater our chance of success. A general goal would be "to heal." A specific goal might be to be able to touch our toes without pain or to lift fifty pounds. Measurable targets let us know when we succeed.

Goals must be attainable—but not too attainable. If we set our goals too high, we invite failure. If we set our goals too low, we won't reach our true potential.

If our goal was to lift fifty pounds in eight weeks, we might begin with a goal of lifting ten pounds in two weeks and progress to lifting twenty-five pounds in four weeks.

Some find it beneficial to actually record goals in some fashion—anything from a diary note to a wall poster. Forms to record and document both long- and short-terms goals and progress are available at www.livingabled.com.

Sometimes it is best to take it one day at a time—not worrying about the future.

Healthy Bodies

Regular physical activity is one of the most important things we can do for our health—physical and mental. Injury, illness, or even most disabilities should not stop us from staying active. We may need to modify what we do, but we want to be doing the most we can.

Staying Active

In 1996 Mile Stojkoski suffered a spinal-cord injury from a motorcycle accident. His accident left him a paraplegic, without the use of his legs. After facing shock and emotional distress he actively worked at his rehabilitation. Stojkoski began competing in sports such as gymnastics, kayaking, ping-pong, soccer, and swimming.

Stojkoski recognized that some others facing such injuries were not always as positive and strong willed as he had been in adapting to injuries and in continuing to live normal lives. Stojkoski became an inspirational speaker and a role model particularly known for competing, using just a regular wheelchair, in cross-country ultra-marathons.

Physical activity increases our energy and stamina, improves our minds, and lengthens our lives. Exercise helps control our weight, fights disease, improves our moods, promotes sleep, and even boosts our sex lives.

It is understandable to want to rest when we are injured or ill. However, we get better faster when we focus on resuming or even increasing our activities. Like professional athletes, we need to get back into the game as quickly as possible.

When we don't exercise regularly we tire more easily and the more easily we tire the less likely we are to exercise. We can break this cycle simply by beginning—and continuing—regular activity.

When we are less active we are more susceptible to minor pains. With nearly any injury or illness, becoming more active will help us. Exercise is an effective antidepressant, comparable to potent antidepressant drugs with far fewer health risks.

If we have not been active for a while we will need to gradually work up to higher levels of activity. Walking or swimming are excellent starts. We all need conditioning, flexibility, and strengthening. Ideally we want to aim for at least thirty minutes of activity every day—but any amount of exercise will be more beneficial to us than no exercise.

Healthy Eating—Diet choices affect our health and weight. Controlling our diets is more effective than any but the most extreme (all day, full-time, Olympic-training-level) workouts.

The food we eat, what and how much, is important to our recovery. Fresh, unprocessed foods help us stay healthy and heal. Highly processed sugars and excessively fatty foods harm us. Sometimes we buy processed foods because they are easy, often cheap, and leave us full. Like choosing excessive medication, they seem to be a quick fix. Like the pharmaceutical industry, the American food industry advertises heavily to convince us to purchase their processed products. Better choices include fresh fruits and vegetables, healthy protein (animal or vegetable), and whole grains.

We need fluids. Our bodies depend on water. Water carries nutrients, flushes out toxins, and provides a hydrated environment for our organs. Healthy adults living in temperate climates need between nine and thirteen cups of water a day depending on their size and activities. We don't have to actually drink all of that; we can get a lot of water through our foods—especially raw fruits and vegetables.

We are better off drinking water than sugary and/or chemical-laden beverages.

Our best current medical recommendations are for us to consume no more than six teaspoons of sugar a day. This equals twenty-four grams. But the average American consumes twenty-two to thirty teaspoons of sugar every day—several times what is recommended. Much of this is hidden in our beverages and processed foods. One bottled fruit drink, store-brand snack cake, or four tablespoons of barbecue sauce typically contain more sugar than our suggested daily limit. Excess sugar contributes to our obesity, diabetes, and other problems.

Of the U.S. population slightly less than a third are considered to be underweight or to have a "normal" healthy weight. Almost exactly a third are considered to be overweight.

And over a third are considered obese—defined by having body mass indexes of 30 or higher. Body mass index (BMI) ratings are calculated on the basis of our height and weight. They are not always the most accurate assessments but they do serve as useful guides. Online BMI calculators are readily available on the Internet. One link is provided in the Internet resources in the back of *Living Abled and Healthy* and is available at www.livingabled.com.

Obesity increases our risk of such diseases as cancer, depression, diabetes, and high blood pressure. Obesity may generate health problems involving our muscles, nerves, tendons, or bones including back pain, joint pain, and carpal tunnel syndrome. It may lead to disability.

Both our eating habits and exercise/activity habits may need to change for us to establish a healthy weight. To lose weight over the long term, in the simplest description, we need to consume fewer calories in what we eat and drink than we burn in our exercise/activities. We need to eat smarter and stay active.

Eating for Recovery—When we are recovering from a muscle injury we need to increase protein intake to offset muscle breakdown. We should divide daily meals into four-to-six smaller portions with complete lean proteins such as are found in lean beef, cottage cheese, fish, poultry, or whey-protein powder. In the early stages of healing we want to also have adequate carbohydrates. After a week or two, however, we need to be cautious that we do not eat too much and gain weight. Healthy choices include beans, fruits, oats and other whole grains, and vegetables. We want to avoid sugars and refined carbohydrates.

There are good fats and bad fats. Omega-3s and monosaturated fats assist in reducing inflammation. These good fats are found in avocados, fatty fish, nuts, olive oil, and flax, pumpkin, sunflower, or sesame seeds. We will be healthier if we avoid the trans fats and saturated fats often found in prepared foods.

Sleep—Sleep is essential to our well-being. Science continues to learn more and more about how sleep restores both our bodies and our minds. Being active during the day will help in our getting enough good sleep at night. We want to go to bed only when we plan to sleep (not to watch television) and avoid stimulants such as coffee in the evening.

Smoking—Sometimes we make choices such as smoking or consuming too much alcohol and/or other drugs. These choices hurt us and slow our recovery.

By now, whatever our personal habits may actually be, we all know that smoking is not good for us. Recent science shows smoking reduces life expectancy, on average, by at least ten years. Those of us who smoke could significantly extend our lives—and live healthier lives— simply by quitting.

What we all might *not* know is that smoking is also a risk factor for certain types of chronic pain, including chronic low-back pain. Smokers with these chronic pains have more severe claims of functional disability, greater depression, and poorer outcomes.

We have many options to help us stop smoking. Using nicotine patches or chewing nicotine gum for a short while are two. Medications can make it easier for us to stop smoking. There are government and other public programs to help us stop smoking. The first step for any of these choices is our commitment to stopping.

Healthy Spirits

Spirit has many different meanings depending on our beliefs. It may reflect existence beyond mind and body. Having a larger perspective may help us to move beyond the physical and mental challenges we face. Some of us may find the concept of spirit in our religious beliefs.

Determination, Faith, and Hope

Bethany Hamilton is now a professional surfer from Kaua'i, Hawai'i. In 2003, at the age of thirteen, Hamilton survived a shark attack in which she lost her left arm. Less than one month after the attack she returned to her board and went surfing. In three months she was again surfing competitively and won her first national title just over a year after her injury. Hamilton shares her experiences, and her faith, in her autobiography Soul Surfer. *Her book was later adapted to become a feature film of the same name. One of her messages is to always strive to be the best at whatever we do. For her and many of us our faith provides strength. It is all perspective. Her acts of courage have become a source of inspiration for many.*

Sometimes we may feel overwhelmed. A healthy spirit will help get us through such dark times. Prayer for ourselves or others is one way many of us seek to support healing. For many of us our faith provides us with purpose and a foundation for resiliency.

What Do We Do?

We take control of our lives and accept responsibility for all aspects of who we are. Healthy minds, bodies, and spirits allow us to experience life more fully and with greater happiness.

3

Our Minds and Our Bodies—
How They Connect

I finally got it.
I was reading and found "A cheerful heart is good
medicine, but a crushed spirit dries up the bones."
I realized I could get past my injury—I just needed to
change my thinking.
That one insight transformed my life.

Challenged and Empowered

Our problems may seem immense to us—and maybe even overpowering. And we may be facing truly serious problems. We might find some perspective by seeing how others with problems just as serious—and often far worse—have faced and overcome their problems.

We may draw inspiration from wounded warriors, military veterans who have suffered severe injuries—including loss of arms or legs or severe spinal-cord injuries—and have faced the horrors of combat. What these men and women have *not* lost is their courage.

Wounded Warrior Amputee Softball Team

The courage of many U.S. wounded warriors is reflected in their Wounded Warrior Amputee Softball Team. Players are young, competitive, athletic veterans and active-duty military who have lost limbs. They include individuals with amputations of an arm, of a leg either below or above the knee, and of both legs below the knees. Their mission is to raise awareness, through

29

exhibition and celebrity softball games, of the sacrifices and resilience of our military and highlight their ability to rise above any challenge. These athletes live out their desires by playing the sport they love. Their motto is "Life Without a Limb is Limitless."

What goes on in our minds—attitudes, beliefs, perceptions, and resiliency—significantly affects what happens in our bodies. Thoughts affect bodies as much—or more—as bodies affect thoughts. Maintaining a strong spirit gives us purpose. Mastering these concepts helps us master our lives.

Our attitudes, beliefs, and perceptions are molded by our experiences and influenced by others. When facing injury or illness we can become empowered or we can become "dis/abled." Sometimes others—for their own sense of control, for greed, for commitment to "standard protocols," or simply for their convenience—will attempt to limit our empowerment and independence.

To better understand how our attitudes, beliefs, perceptions, and resiliency shape who we are, we need to focus on our mind-body connection. Body, mind, and spirit are all connected. Changing any part of our reality affects all of our reality.

When we are physically hurt we have changed our body. Any pain we feel may be driven by local nerves but our perception of that pain takes place in our brain. If our brain experiences intense pain, or any pain for a long time, or, worst of all, intense pain for a long time, our brain will actually, scientifically measurably, change. As our brain changes, changes in our body will also occur. Such changes may also affect our emotions and spirit.

But one of the most natural things our bodies do is to heal. While our bodies can fix many of our injuries they cannot fix them all. Through evolution we have lost our ability to re-grow missing limbs, major nerves, or organs—although promising research indicates we may someday in the future regain some of this ability with the help of medical science. Today our most successful healing comes when we pay attention to *all* of what makes us who we are.

To better understand how body, mind, and spirit are connected we need look no further than at those who, despite significant physical challenges, live joyful and productive lives. Unfortunately, at the same time, we need to also look at those who have become trapped by "needless disability." We must look at what causes some of us to take a disabling path while others of us, facing similar or worse problems, choose an empowering path.

When we cannot control and do not understand what is happening to us, we can become confused, depressed, and scared. *Understanding* improves our resilience and helps us successfully cope with what we may not be able to control. Understanding can help us move past what we may first see as impossible barriers. Understanding can also provide clarity to navigate the complex maze of government, health, insurance, and legal systems we may face.

Sometimes, when we become injured or ill, some of us will use our difficulty to reinvent ourselves and live beyond our challenges. Rather than complaining or wallowing in self-pity we will use our challenges as a chance for growth. It is easy to focus on our loss, pain, or other symptoms—but we always have choices.

When we are not who we were, we can become who we will be. We need never see ourselves as "disabled," only "differently abled." We can focus on what we can become. We can learn from others who fully embrace life despite what some might see as impossible barriers.

Courage

A classic scene from the 2012 film Battleship *shows a legless, wounded army veteran dragging himself up a mountain to battle aliens invading earth. Our wounded hero becomes largely responsible for saving the world.*

Obviously this is a movie fantasy—but the star of this movie was U.S. Army Colonel Gregory D. Gadson and his real-life story may be even more inspirational than the movie. Gadson is a double amputee who, in 2007 in Iraq, lost both legs above the knees to a roadside bomb. In 2009 he became the first person to use the then-most-current-version of powered prosthetic knees featuring artificial intelligence and sensor technology making it possible for above-the-knee amputees to walk with increased confidence and a more natural gait.

This war veteran went back to school after his injury and earned a master's degree and was awarded an additional honorary degree. Gadson became an honorary co-captain of the New York Giants football team after sharing a motivational pep talk. While no one can say with certainty the effects of Gadson's motivation, following his talk the Giants began a ten-game winning streak culminating with the 2007 Super Bowl championship. After acting in Battleship, Gadson was still on active duty in 2013.

Gadson has said, simply, "I couldn't stand quitting. I couldn't stand the silence. I couldn't stand giving up."

Those of us who respond to challenges by demanding empowerment share common beliefs focusing on moving beyond our physical or psychological limitations. We often experience joyful and productive lives. Many times we turn limitations into strengths.

Frequently we describe our focus with such words as: commitment, confidence, courage, determination, faith, hope, optimism, purpose, resiliency, spirit, and vision.

Needlessly Disabled

"Needlessly disabled" is a term describing those of us who come to believe ourselves disabled, or act as if we are disabled, when there is little medical evidence supporting this conclusion. Sometimes we have been victimized by various systems simply following their "path of least resistance." Sometimes it becomes less work for others to label us disabled than it would be for them to provide us support for our enablement. Sometimes we have been victimized by others who profit from our disability.

There may be a complex web of participants in our disabling process. It may start with poor parenting or abuse and may be aided by learned expectations of entitlement versus expectations of responsibility. Often it may involve our lacking training in effective coping skills.

Whatever outside factors may be driving us toward needless disablement, we need to recognize our independence and responsibility. We need to make the decisions leading us to enabled lives focused on improving and regaining our health and function.

John is an active, energetic twenty-year-old who falls off of a ladder at work, immediately feels his low-back begin to tighten and hurt, and is taken to the emergency room. There a spinal x-ray reveals an injury John is told is a "pars interarticularis" spine fracture.

As John tries to make sense of this confusing term, and what it means to him, he remembers a cousin who fractured his spine and became paralyzed below his waist. Understandably, John begins to worry.

John goes to a "pain clinic" doctor who gives him a narcotic opioid for his pain. The doctor tells John he must be careful not to do anything that might worsen his injury or cause more problems. The doctor tells John that he will need to see a doctor regularly, possibly for the rest of his life.

This doctor has magnified John's natural fears by encouraging him to believe that if he participates in any activity—sports or at his job— he will worsen his injury.

Other than visiting his doctor on alternate weeks, John stops all of his activities and spends his days resting; he is convinced he is disabled for life. He is bored, discouraged, and realizes he now tires easily. He gains weight and sees himself as less of a person than he had been before his accident.

A year later, at the suggestion of a good friend, John sees a different doctor.

The new doctor is compassionate and listens to John's fears. His new doctor reassures John that his injury is common and rarely causes long-term problems. John's new doctor tells him that his injury is also called "lumbar spondylolysis" and is a common cause of low-back pain in adolescent athletes. John's injury is reported in roughly 30 percent of adolescents actively participating in sports.

John begins a program of physical conditioning. Ten weeks later John is again enjoying his sports and has returned to working.

Based mostly upon what his first doctor had told him, and helped along by memories of his cousin, John believed he had fractured his back and could easily become paralyzed. Believing that, he allowed fear to dominate his life, became inactive, and lost his athletic conditioning.

When more realistically informed of how common his injury was and how unlikely it was to cause him further problems, John's beliefs changed. With just some conditioning needed for his year of inactivity, he reclaimed his life.

Self-descriptions from those of us challenged and empowered are different from self-descriptions from those of us needlessly disabled. To help us better avoid becoming trapped by false labels, we can learn from the stories of others tragically caught in such a downward spiral.

Doctors who see the "needlessly disabled" cannot find any identifiable physiologic reasons for their disability. Physical examinations typically show nothing unusual. If we cling to beliefs of disability while confronting a lack of identifiable medical causes, we may become angry. We may focus on what we cannot do—rather than on what we can do—and we may feel trapped. Understanding how this has happened to others can help us get past our feelings of being trapped.

How We're All Different

Our bodies, minds, and spirits determine who we are. They are our "empowerment" or our "needless disability."

Our bodies vary, reflecting our genetic heritages, nutrition (including our early nutrition and even that of our parents), environmental exposures, injuries and illnesses, and lifestyle choices. Our post-childhood body changes often reflect choices regarding alcohol, tobacco, and other drugs; eating habits; and physical activity.

Our minds shape how we deal with stress (from both our normal daily lives and from major life changes). Our minds identify the differences between what is normal, such as discomfort or feeling tired, and what is not normal, such as injury or illness. Partially we will reflect how we have seen others deal with potentially disabling events. Some of us cope with injury, illness, stress, and disability better than others. Some of us are more resilient in dealing with life's challenges.

Our spirits can be said to reflect who we are beyond our physical bodies and our minds. Spirit may be called our essence of meaning or soul. Our bodies and minds may be strengthened by a spirit of empowerment.

When we are happy and satisfied with our lives and our jobs we better deal with health challenges. Our personalities, mental toughness, and the presence or absence of prior mental problems all affect how we react to new problems. Perceptions of gain, financial or otherwise, may also affect how we react.

We can contrast attributes of those of us who are "challenged and empowered" with those of us who have become "needlessly disabled" in the following table and self-assessment exercise. While the named characteristics may describe many of us, there is no possible list that could define all of our reactions. The more we reflect positive responses the more likely we are to experience "abled" and healthy lives.

Challenged and Empowered versus Needlessly Disabled

	Challenged & Empowered	Needlessly Disabled
Behavior	Cheerful	Depressed
Catastrophizes	Rarely	Often
Confidence	Strong	Weak
Coping skills	Strong	Weak
Emotions	Gratitude	Anger
Emphasizes	Strength	Weakness
Excuses	Few	Many
Fear	Rarely	Often
Focus	Function	Symptoms
Health knowledge	High	Low
Honesty	Yes	Maybe
Hope	Often	Rarely
Humor	Often	Rarely
Litigates	Rarely	Often
Perceives problems	Challenges/ opportunities	Barriers
Perspective	Positive (Optimistic)	Negative (Pessimistic)
Physically	Active	Inactive
Reactions	Forgiveness	Blame
Relationships	Independent	Dependent
Resiliency	Strong	Weak
Responsibility	Self	Others

A Self-Assessment of Personality Characteristics

Check those statements that generally apply:

- Others describe me as "cheerful."
- I expect "best case" outcomes, not "worst case" outcomes.
- I am confident about finding my way through life.
- I have strong coping skills.
- I focus on my strengths rather than on my weaknesses.
- I rarely make excuses.
- I am usually fearless.
- I experience gratitude more often than I experience anger.
- I focus on my ability to function rather than on my symptoms.
- I am knowledgeable about my health.
- I am honest.
- I am hopeful.
- I have a good sense of humor.
- I try to avoid litigation and lawyers.
- I am optimistic.
- I am active.
- I see problems as challenges rather than as barriers.
- I am forgiving.
- I am independent.
- I am self-responsible.
- I am resilient.

The more of these statements we can claim as personal truths the more likely we are to do well. For those statements we could not now claim as personal truths, we should consider how we might change our lives so we can someday soon claim them as our own.

Mind-Changing Experiences

Our perception of pain is in our brains. We talk about having pains in specific parts of our bodies, such as backs, necks, or shoulders, but the reality is that all of our pains are actually experienced in our brains.

Over the years we can see our bodies change—sometimes for better, sometimes for worse. Brains also change. Not only do we face gradual transitions as we age but our brains also undergo dynamic and rapid adaptation throughout our lives.

Beliefs and experiences physically alter our brains. Our beliefs and experiences change who we are. Our brains and nervous systems adapt, both structurally and functionally, to our environment. We call this ability of our brains to constantly change "neuroplasticity."

Changes in our brains and nervous systems come most often from repeated activities, doing the same thing over and over. This is good news. Even as adults our brains remain adaptive and "plastic." Experience and practice produces the "muscle memory" of athletes and the playing ability of musicians.

We see positive changes when we are determined to repeatedly practice our therapies even when we are recovering from an injury or illness that left us with brain damage. Such changes are seen and documented by doctors using brain-imaging tools. Not all of our changes are always for the better. Doctors also see and document brain changes in those of us who face chronic pain or become addicted to drugs.

Scientific advances in neuro-imaging and neurophysiology have brought us these insights. Brain SPECT (Single Photon Emission Computed Tomography) and fMRI (functional Magnetic Resonance Imaging) provide real-time pictures of blood flow and activity patterns in our brains.

Areas of our brains, commonly called the "pain matrix," may show abnormalities on imaging studies of those experiencing chronic pain. The same areas will be affected even when pain comes from different parts of our bodies or comes from different causes—even emotional pain.

Our brain connections, called synapses, change to connect our symptoms (sensations) with what we come to believe about our symptoms—beliefs usually based on the diagnosis we have been given by our doctor. Belief in our diagnosis and focus on our experience with our injury may actually lead to additional or more intense symptoms.

Sometimes others try to change our beliefs to fit their own purposes. Sometimes this is blatant but often this may be exceptionally subtle and we may not even see it happening.

If we focus less on our symptoms, our brains are capable of changing back to much like they were before we were injured. Who we believe ourselves to be largely defines who we are.

Learned Helplessness

Some of us are better at handling added stress; we are more resilient. Others of us are not as resilient and we may experience "learned helplessness."

Mary and David are middle-aged friends working for the same employer. Mary enjoys athletic pursuits including tennis and running while David prefers to take it easy when not working.

Mary notices some neck pain one day and sees a sports-medicine doctor, Dr. Taylor. Dr. Taylor reassures Mary that her sort of neck pain is common, that no immediate testing is needed, and that there is no immediate need for extensive treatment. Mary is told to do some stretching exercises and take some over-the-counter ibuprofen for a couple of days. Her pain goes away.

David develops a sudden neck pain while at work and goes to the hospital emergency room. Because the emergency room is already overloaded with serious trauma cases, the emergency doctor refers David to Dr. Miller at the Injury Treatment Center.

Dr. Miller makes most of his income from treating non-life-threatening vehicle accidents and workers' compensation patients. His office is not a trauma center for serious injuries. The more Dr. Miller does, the more money he makes. His income is generated by fees for examinations and other office visits, various tests, a variety of treatments (some of which may be questionable), and payments for medications and devices dispensed directly from his office (often at several times the price they might be purchased elsewhere). Dr. Miller frequently finds the problems of the patients he examines are caused by an accident- or work-related injury (guaranteeing payment).

David is advised to "rest" and prescribed a narcotic opioid pain medicine. David is particularly concerned when an immediately ordered MRI scan of his spine reveals degenerative disc disease. This is a diagnosis that would be likely from MRI scans of most middle-aged spines—probably including Mary's. However, Dr. Miller explains this as a serious finding requiring ongoing treatment, which Dr. Miller will be happy to provide. All of these elements focus David on his symptoms—and may lead to even greater problems.

While resting at home David watches television and sees ads for lawyers who will represent injury victims and get them "fair" compensation settlements. Already confused by his opioid medication and the injury-treatment process, David contacts Lawyer Baker. Lawyer Baker explains that he will fight for David and will not charge David for his services unless he gets David compensation.

Lawyer Baker advises David to follow the guidance of Dr. Miller, with whom he has worked many times in the past, and especially to follow Dr. Miller's advice to avoid being physically active or returning to his job—these "dangerous" undertakings could reduce the amount of David's potential compensation. Lawyer Baker does not mention to David that he is not overly concerned regarding possibly unnecessary care or high bills since these increase the value of the case and, if favorably settled, his fees.

David is still confused. However, as he is living pretty much on his own, he is happy to have the emotional support of both Dr. Miller and Lawyer Baker. Besides David never cared much for his boss—and his boss has not even called to see how David is feeling.

David's symptoms have been reinforced by the labels assigned by Dr. Miller and reinforced by Lawyer Baker; David now recognizes he is a victim. He is confused and he does not understand what is happening. He becomes angry.

Matters get worse when David's company's insurance claims adjuster questions him, and a lawyer representing the insurance company raises doubts about his complaints. David is then seen by independent medical evaluators who appear not to believe he is injured. Dr. Miller comforts David and advises him that such doctors just work for the insurance companies and that Dr. Miller will continue to take good care of him.

David begins a downward spiral of increasing pain, confusion, loss of conditioning, and anger. He can't understand why his luck has been so bad.

Mary's doctor did not do immediate extensive testing. He reassured Mary and focused her on her function. As well as continuing at her job, Mary has returned to playing sports.

As David becomes entangled in more testing and more treatment and as his confusing legal case demands more of his attention and generates ever-more anger, David sinks deeper into his role of victim. The neural connections in David's brain reinforcing this role continue to strengthen.

David becomes upset when Mary suggests Dr. Miller and Lawyer Baker may not really be concerned with David's well-being. Mary suggests they may just be using David for their own financial gain.

Although David did not like his boss, he misses his coworkers. He has now been away from his job for three months. David hopes his settlement will be large because he knows he will have to live with his degenerative disc disease for the rest of his life.

David is now facing a difficult future. He believes himself disabled. If nothing else, his belief alone will likely make this true. For those of us who do not return to our jobs in three-to-six months, the probability of our eventual return is halved. If we do not return to our jobs, our risks for illness and early death increase.

Whatever physical problems David may face, those problems have now been made worse by psychological issues. Neuroplasticity has likely led to harmful changes in David's brain so his pain may be worse and last longer—maybe for the rest of his life. All of this is reversible—it just takes a change in perspective. More importantly, it was preventable.

Despite likely having no significant differences in their problems, David was not as resilient as Mary. He learned to become helpless. Our resiliency to stressors is influenced—but not controlled—by our prior lifetime experiences. When we accept believing we cannot cope, we have "learned helplessness." We stop seeking positive rewards and fail to take advantage of all possible opportunities to avoid bad outcomes. We have given up our freedoms and our independence.

Depression and other mental problems often stem from believing we have no control over our lives. The more we view our lives as being under our control, the less we stress and the more hope we have for improving our lives.

Understanding neuroplasticity helps us understand why Mary continued at her job and returned to her sports while David became disabled. If we need to prove we have problems or that someone else is responsible for our problems, we stay focused on our problems. When we do not understand what caused our problems we often worry and focus on our symptoms.

Extensive medical testing and extended treatments reinforce our belief of serious problems. The more our doctors do for us the more we may believe we have serious problems.

If our problems are blamed on an injury for which we may receive financial compensation, the design of the insurance and legal systems in the United States (and many other places) may cause others to act in ways that are not ultimately in our best interest. We may come to believe we are more injured, ill, or disabled than we actually are. These beliefs may alter our brains and we may experience more pain, become less independent, and face risks from unnecessary drugs and treatment.

Injuries in workplace settings, or from personal injuries such as vehicle accidents, have been scientifically documented to have dramatically worse outcomes than similar accidents from sports injuries.

What Do We Do?

We want to learn from those we see who are "challenged and empowered" and avoid being trapped into "needless disability." We want to maintain control and independence and always approach life with positive attitudes.

4

What Do We Mean?

Everything the doctors said just confused me more.
They kept talking some foreign language. Only after
a nurse explained what was going on did it begin to
make some sense.
I finally figured out that some of my treatments were
actually causing some of my problems.
Now I tell my doctors that nothing happens unless I
understand what is happening—both what benefits I
am supposed to be getting and what side effects I may
suffer. I demand they give me scientific, evidence-
based, reasons for any recommendations.
Slowly I am starting to feel better.

Foreign Lands

When we travel to foreign lands, the more we learn about the people who live there the better we will be able to understand those we meet. For most of us, medicine and law are foreign lands. We need to understand these cultures and their "magic" words. Words can be powerful. If we fail to learn enough to understand important words from these cultures, we may become confused, lost. If we use the words of these cultures without fully understanding those words, we may be saying things we do not really mean. Both not understanding what is being said to us and our own use of words without full and accurate understanding may cause us real problems.

Disease, Disorder, Injury, Illness, and Syndrome

We want to understand what is meant by "disease," "disorder," "injury," "illness," and "syndrome." We may easily confuse these terms and mislead others or even ourselves. Problems labeled as disease may not really be "diseases"—for example, degenerative disk disease. "Injuries" and "syndromes" may be mislabeled. An "illness" may not reflect a true physical problem.

Disease is an abnormal condition affecting our body. Disease may cause distress, dysfunction, pain, or even death. Usually our doctors can identify something specifically wrong—an objectively definable medical abnormality. Diseases may affect us physically and emotionally. Chronic diseases may alter our perspective on life. We may have heart disease and our response may be to become less active. Becoming less active may lead to our gaining weight and other problems including depression.

Jack is sixty years old and experiences shoulder pain. He sees Dr. Wilson who orders an MRI scan of his shoulder. The scan reveals degenerative processes involving Jack's rotator cuff—the muscles and tendons surrounding Jack's shoulder. The scan also shows a partial tear of one of these structures. Dr. Wilson explains to Jack that these findings show he has a significant disease and needs surgery.

Jack's damaged rotator cuff and the finding of the tear may not be the cause of Jack's pain. Such changes are often seen as we age. Jack has been told he has a disease—this may not be true. Jack's scan may simply be showing changes commonly associated with aging.

Sometimes (sometimes even with the help of our doctors) we confuse the normal effects of aging with disease. Frequently, as we age, our hair turns gray or we lose some or all of it—this is not a disease.

Spines also age and discs (the shock-absorbing structures between the vertebrae bones in our spine) will often lose fluid, become thinner, and possibly bulge, crack, fragment, or tear. These changes occur over time and are largely a result of genetics. Such changes are found in four out of ten of us over thirty-five and in almost all of us over fifty. If we are over fifty and our back pain causes us to have spinal x-rays taken, those x-rays will almost always show disk degeneration. Often this is *not* the cause of our back pain. Acute trauma, such as a fall or sudden heavy lifting, may worsen our problems or cause a tear; however the underlying disc degeneration itself is something that occurs over time.

Most of the time doctors cannot define the actual cause of back pain.

It simply is. Doctors identify this as "non-specific low-back pain"—but putting a name on pain does not mean doctors will always, or even often, have solutions.

A *disorder* is a functional abnormality or disturbance. It is something damaging our ability to function. Doctors may categorize medical disorders into emotional and behavioral disorders, functional disorders, genetic disorders, mental disorders, or physical disorders. Sometimes disorders may be difficult to categorize.

Emotional and behavioral disorders may be diagnosed in children and are often difficult to define. In some cases these diagnoses are considered subjective—that is, they are the *opinion* of the examining doctor and cannot be identified by objective measures. Commonly these disorders are characterized by "out of control" aggressive behaviors expressed outwardly, or by being socially withdrawn, or by infrequent but serious symptoms of psychiatric disorders such as schizophrenia.

Functional disorders are conditions where we display symptoms without contemporary medical science being able to detect any evidence of physical disease. These may also be referred to as medically unexplained symptoms. Chronic fatigue syndrome (associated with prolonged and profound fatigue) and irritable bowel syndrome (associated with abdominal pain and cramping and changes in our bowel movements) are examples. Specific causes of functional disorders are currently unknown. Having a functional disorder does not mean we are making up our symptoms, it only means that contemporary medical science cannot explain why we have our symptoms.

Genetic disorders are caused by abnormalities in genes or chromosomes. These disorders may be complex and associated with the effects from multiple genes in combination with our environmental and lifestyle factors. Certain cancers could be examples of genetic disorders.

Mental disorders are psychological patterns resulting in identifiable behaviors typically associated with our distress or disability. According to the World Health Organization over a third of us in most countries at some time in our lives report problems meeting the criteria for a diagnosis of a mental disorder. Our being diagnosed as having a mental disorder should not cause us to be stigmatized or face discrimination. Our disorder may be a problem but it is not who we are.

Physical disorders are common. Even when contemporary medical science cannot provide explanations, such as for many of our back pains, physical disorders are generally assumed to have physical causes.

Injury refers to physical damage to some part of the body. Injuries may be acute (sudden and severe) or chronic (resulting from long-term activities). We want to distinguish actual damage caused by an injury from our experience of a symptom. Sometimes our problem may be caused by a specific event. Other times our problem may simply be caused by our living longer.

Illness is the subjective feeling of being unwell. We perceive it as a state of poor health. When health is defined as "complete physical, mental, and social well-being," being ill is our personal experience of not feeling right.

Jessica feels ill, she looks ill, and everyone treats her as if she is ill. Jessica needs to be cared for.

Jessica may be ill but she may have nothing physically wrong with her. Illness is recognized as a disease only when a physical process is detected. We may feel ill and we may have undeniable symptoms but this does not necessarily mean we have a measureable physical problem. On the other hand, we may actually have a serious disease without our being "ill." We could have high blood pressure (hypertension) or other problems—even some early-stage cancers—and have no easily recognizable symptoms.

Illness is culturally defined and socially sanctioned. Each culture defines what it means to be ill and this varies from one culture to another. Different societies adopt certain rules of behavior about being ill and whether being ill does or does not mean we need to be cared for and/or freed of our usual responsibilities. If we think we are ill, if we act as if we are ill, and if our culture and society treats us as if we are ill, then we are ill. In American society the phrase of "I feel ill" is a common expression when we have encountered some shocking situation.

Syndrome refers to a collection of certain clinically recognizable features that may include symptoms (sensations we report), signs (objective observations by others), or phenomena (a fact or event which may be scientifically described or explained). Specific syndromes usually include certain essential characteristics. Some syndromes, such

∕

as carpal tunnel (compression of the median nerves in our wrists), are well-defined. Others, such as chronic fatigue syndrome or complex regional pain syndrome, however, currently lack generally accepted and detailed definitions and can be more controversial diagnoses.

We want our doctors to accurately diagnose any disease, disorder, injury, illness, or syndrome. If our diagnosis is serious, it is almost always worth our time and expense to seek a second qualified opinion before proceeding with dangerous medications or extensive therapies. If doctors disagree on our diagnosis, we may need to seek more than two consultations to feel comfortable with a conclusion. We need to know as best as we can that whatever label given to our complaint is accurate.

When we feel ill we need to understand that we may not necessarily have an identifiable physical or mental problem. We must also recognize that not all injury or illness is caused by a specific event. Symptoms or disease may simply occur as a part of life with no currently identifiable cause. If our doctor tells us we have a "syndrome," we should demand a detailed and thorough explanation of what is meant.

Pains, Signs, and Symptoms

Pain is defined by the International Association for the Study of Pain as an "unpleasant sensory and emotional experience associated with actual or potential tissue damage, or described in terms of such damage." In the United States pain is our most common reason for seeing our doctor.

Pain is "subjective," meaning it is something we experience and we may describe to others but not something objectively measureable by someone else.

If we complain of pain we will commonly be asked to describe our pain on a scale of zero (no pain) to ten (our worst imaginable pain)—but doctors have no device or instrument to independently measure our pain. We each have our own perception of what our "ten" pain may be. As our lives change we may come to redefine what a pain of "ten" means to us.

A medical *sign* is an objective indication of some medical fact doctors may detect during our examination or from clinical studies. Objective indications may be independently verified by multiple doctors.

"Signs" are different from "findings." Many items noted as

examination "findings" are not objective—they depend on our reporting. Our reports of experiencing tenderness or our reports of other sensations are examples. Other findings by our doctors, such as measurements of range of motion or strength, may be consciously or unconsciously influenced by our behavior. Because of pain or our fear of pain we may demonstrate less motion or strength than we could actually achieve.

Michael is in his car and stopped for a red light when his car is struck from behind. The other vehicle does not appear to have been going fast and there is no significant damage to the bumpers of either car. Still, Michael's neck feels sore. He goes to an injury clinic and is diagnosed as suffering from "whiplash." As Michael continues to see his doctor over months for his whiplash, his neck pain continues and his doctor reports that Michael has significant findings of tenderness.

Michael has a symptom—he has pain. Michael's doctor's report of a finding of "tenderness" is based on what Michael tells his doctor. It is how Michael feels when he is touched, not something Michael's doctor can identify or measure without Michael's input.

A *symptom* is a sensation departing from our normal function or feeling which we identify. Symptoms may be acute or chronic. They may indicate disease or abnormality—or not. Symptoms are sensations reaching our awareness and becoming bothersome or of concern.

Symptoms such as headaches, other pains, or fatigue may suggest we may have a disease or abnormality—or not. Symptoms cannot always be explained by any currently measurable underlying changes in our physiology.

Many symptoms may be perfectly normal and related to our normal realities. If we become active in ways we haven't been before, or haven't been for a long time, experiencing some minor pain or stiffness over following days could be perfectly normal. This is common when we return to an activity we once did regularly but have not done for years or decades. Our minds may remember a level of capability we have not maintained in our bodies.

Nonspecific symptoms are symptoms we experience but do not, as best as current medicine can tell, indicate a specific disease process or involve a specific aspect of our body. Again, our symptoms could be clinical manifestations of an undiagnosed disease or they could just result from our normal activities and not be associated with any identifiable disease. Feeling tired is a symptom of many physiological and psychological conditions—but it is also a normal, healthy reaction after exerting ourselves or at the end of a long day.

Awareness of symptoms may also relate to psychological factors including our moods, perceptions, and thoughts. When we are anxious or if we become particularly focused on our body's sensations, we are more likely to identify symptoms. Often symptoms we have not even noticed during the course of our day may reach our consciousness only after we have stopped our activities and are resting and trying to sleep.

Subjective experiences are influenced by our attitudes, beliefs, biases, emotions, and/or prejudices. All of these internal factors may also be influenced by the attitudes, beliefs, biases, emotions, and/or prejudices of others. Most of us have seen small children hurt themselves in some minor way and show little reaction—until some nearby adult becomes overly excited and the child begins to wail.

Michael's neck pain, described earlier, may be another example. Michael could have seen his regular doctor. That doctor might have told Michael he suffered a minor strain, which could be helped by some acetaminophen (commonly sold as Tylenol®) or ibuprofen (commonly sold as Advil® or Motrin®) and would likely go away in a few days or a week at most.

Or the doctor Michael saw at the injury clinic may have helped Michael create a belief that his neck pain is the result of a serious problem and needs extensive (and costly) treatment.

Michael may then find a lawyer who may reinforce Michael's belief he has had a serious injury.

In either case, Michael's perception of his pain would have been influenced by a doctor (and possibly also by a lawyer). Michael, however, will likely never know how he has been influenced.

Symptoms without signs typically do not reflect significant physical problems. If we have symptoms such as pain, and competent doctors are unable to find evidence of a disease, it is less likely we have a significant physical problem.

Placebo Effect

When we consider the effectiveness of various treatments, we need to understand what is meant by the "placebo effect." "Placebo" is a Latin word meaning "I shall please." It refers to inert or innocuous substances or other treatments often used as test references in scientific studies. Historically this has frequently been a "sugar pill" looking the same as other pills carrying active medications being studied. Sometimes doctors may deliberately prescribe placebos for psychological purposes.

If we believe our problems are being treated we may often have a perceived or actual improvement in our condition. As we discussed earlier, the mind-body connection is strong. This may be true even if the treatments have no physiological basis. This is known as the "placebo effect." Many of our positive encounters with doctors have therapeutic value because of the placebo effect. This is particularly true when doctors are caring and reassuring, even when they do not prescribe a specific treatment. We go to our doctors, share our concerns, they empathize, and often we feel better when we leave their offices.

Placebo effects are self-fulfilling expectations that our treatments will improve our condition. Placebo treatments may cause us actual physiological changes—they may result in real physical changes to our bodies. Placebos appear to work most effectively with our subjective conditions such as depression or pain.

If we have a compassionate doctor providing us medications or treatments we may find our problem improving. Sometimes this improvement may not be from the physiological component of medications or treatments but from our own expectations. This improvement may be from the placebo effect or just from our normal recovery from an injury or illness that would have occurred without any treatment.

Poor expectations may similarly produce poor results. "Nocebo" is the contrasting Latin for "I will harm." Those of us with chronic pain will often have seen many doctors and tried many treatments without success. We may approach a new provider with all of our negative experiences and expect nothing will work for us. If this is what we believe when we are given a new medication or treatment, we should not be surprised to find our new medication or treatment is not helpful.

Evidence-Based Medicine

When doctors offer us a conclusion or recommendation—whether about our diagnosis, what caused our problem, or ordering tests or treatments—we want to believe they have solid reasons. We want our medical care to be based on the best available evidence, identified by scientific method, for clinical decision-making. This process is known as "evidence-based medicine."

Evidence-based medicine requires that the best and most current medical science be applied to our specific situation. It means that we receive care based on what has been *demonstrated* to work, not what our doctors *think* might work. Evidence-based medicine is never based on personal opinions or anecdotal evidence; it is based on the best and most current scientific information.

Evidence-based medicine is an important principle. We want to understand and use this term and require it for all decisions concerning our care. Evidence-based medicine will assess the strength of scientific evidence for both the benefits and the risks of any diagnostic testing or treatments proposed for us.

Evidence is usually drawn from systematic reviews of current medical literature identifying effective care. Evidence-based medicine categorizes and evaluates clinical evidence. The strongest evidence for specific care comes from randomized, triple-blind, placebo-controlled trials. These studies involve multiple steps to avoid any individuals' preferences or prior expectations affecting trial outcomes.

There is both the science and an "art" of medicine. The art of medicine may reflect subconsciously achieved decisions generated with minimal information using substantial pattern recognition guided by significant personal experience. However, decisions based on personal experience are not as reliable as decisions based on our best scientific evidence. The art of medicine is best reflected when using evidence-based medicine as guidelines adapted to our unique situations. Sometimes medical "arts" may also offer placebo benefits contributing to our healing.

Individual case reports, unsupported "expert" opinions, and patient testimonials are *not* evidence-based medicine. If friends suggest "You should try this because it worked for me" or doctors begin with "In my opinion...," we must be skeptical.

Evidence-based medicine has roots in both ancient and medieval medicine but evolved as a modern practice largely from the work beginning in 1972 by the late British epidemiologist Archie Cochrane (1909–1988). His initial efforts have been further developed and systematized by universities around the world. An international network known as the Cochrane Collaboration now involves over twenty-eight thousand individuals from over one hundred countries.

The Cochrane Collaboration website (www.cochrane.org) and other evidence-based websites provide significant resources to help us determine the most current medical science on a broad range of issues. Our doctors may not always be familiar with the most current science for all possible medical issues. They face demanding schedules and busy lives and medical science is always evolving.

Commonly used Internet search engines rank responses largely on the frequency of access or references to specific sites—and even sometimes by payments—and use search algorithms (sets of rules for solving problems) subject to deliberate manipulation. Accurate scientific information may easily be lost behind better publicized or better financed but biased websites. Many websites highly ranked by Internet search engines display inaccurate information.

Findings from the most current evidence-based medicine may be gathered by groups or associations of medical specialists focusing on a specific medical area or problem. After review of these scientific studies and acceptance by these groups or associations, such findings may be expressed in treatment or practice "guidelines." Guidelines serve to summarize scientific results and provide recommendations for appropriate diagnostic studies and/or treatments. We may expect our doctors to apply these guidelines to our specific situations.

We want to ask our doctors about the evidence-based medicine that supports their recommendations. A list of evidence-based medical websites may be found in the back of *Living Abled and Healthy* and is available at www.livingabled.com.

Shared Decision-Making

"Shared decision-making" is a collaborative process allowing us to participate with our providers in making healthcare decisions. Ideally this involves the practical application of evidence-based medicine—taking into account the best scientific evidence as well as our values and preferences. This honors both our right to always be fully informed and our providers' expert knowledge.

Being informed reflects that we always have choices, there are always options, and there are always both benefits and risks for all options. At times there will be strong evidence supporting a specific treatment program—at other times evidence may support more than one approach or not particularly favor any one approach over others. In our determining what we will do we need to recognize our values and life circumstances.

We always want to remember that we are in control of our bodies and that our control should be limited only by how much we understand. Decision-making concerning our healthcare should be shared; we need a partnership. The more we learn about our medical issues the more we may expect to control and accept responsibility for our care. The less we understand about our medical issues the more we are forced to accept our doctors' suggestions on faith.

Iatrogenesis

While the word "iatrogenesis" originally referred to both good and bad effects *introduced* by doctors' diagnostic procedures or medical treatments; we now almost always use the word to refer to bad effects. Iatrogenesis now commonly describes the unintended creation of a disease or illness through our medical treatment or procedures. The importance of this term is that it is describing a problem we did *not* have *before* our interaction with our healthcare providers.

Our healthcare may sometimes lead us to needless complications, injury, illness, disability, or even death. The causes of iatrogenic problems include adverse effects of treatment, ignorance, inappropriate financial rewards, and negligence. Iatrogenesis is estimated to cause over two hundred thousand deaths a year in the United States.

We are far more likely to die as a result of iatrogenesis than from a vehicle accident or other trauma. Many of us frequently worry about dying in a vehicle crash. Yet we are almost seven times more likely to die from iatrogenic problems—and few of us worry about these.

Contemporary U.S. medical practice and reimbursement systems generally pressure our doctors to quickly "label" us with a diagnosis. If our doctor generates a wrong diagnosis, not only will we likely get the wrong treatment but we are also likely to come to believe and behave as if our diagnosis was accurate.

Financial incentives drive many doctors to keep visits as short as possible. Rather than taking the time needed to understand us and our stories, doctors may rely upon extensive testing and/or excessive medication. Time pressures encourage some doctors to quickly write prescriptions rather than more slowly inform us about how we may best deal with our concerns.

Influenced by the drug advertising we hear and see almost everywhere in the United States and by our rushed doctors, we may develop our own expectations of getting prescription medications. Most doctors are paid more for medical procedures than for providing us with critical medical information. This encourages care through medications and medical procedures—and all medications and medical procedures have associated risks.

Causation

In many disability/injury/illness-compensation systems it is essential for doctors to identify the cause of our problem to determine whether it is "compensable" (whether our medical care or other claims ought to be paid by an employer or insurer). Vehicle-accident compensation only covers payments if the problem came from a specific vehicle accident. Workers' compensation only covers payments if the condition "arose out of and in the course of" our work activities; this generally means that something about our work caused our problem and this occurred while at work. Identifications of causation from legal perspectives may differ from identifications of causation from medical perspectives.

In assessing causation our doctors need to express opinions to a "reasonable degree of medical probability." This means there must be more than a 50 percent likelihood that our doctors' opinions are accurate. This is more than a 50/50 coin-toss likelihood—but anything even just barely better than that 50/50 coin-toss likelihood counts. Our doctors must determine if the problems we are experiencing can be linked, with that "reasonable degree of medical probability," to a specific cause.

Usually what caused our problem will not change how we are treated. Most doctors are not specifically trained in assessing causation. Because our treatments focus on our problems and not on their causes, the study of "causation" is not a major element of most medical training.

This evaluation of causation will, however, be a critical issue if we make a compensation claim. The potential compensation payer may want to deny any connection between our problem and whatever situation (accident, environment, work, etc.) for which that payer may be responsible. We, with our doctors (who will want to be paid for their services), and any lawyers we may involve, may try to prove that connection.

If we are refused compensation for a problem for which a potential payer actually *is* responsible we are being deprived of compensation that is rightfully ours.

On the other hand, if we are seeking compensation for a problem for which a potential payer is *not* actually responsible, not only are we doing something which may be both illegal and morally wrong, we are putting our health at risk. Medical studies show that if our problems are "compensable," often we will not have as good a health outcome as when our problems are "non-compensable."

Causation determination is usually simple for sudden and severe problems such as when we have a broken bone. It will be much more challenging for our chronic problems. But even for initially sudden and severe problems such as those caused by a vehicle accident, it may not be easy for us or for others to determine if that initial event is continuing to cause us problems over time.

When we are contesting a compensation claim our memories of how we were before that initial event may not be as clear as we would like them to be or as clear as they would be if we were not contesting the compensation claim. Sometimes we may ignore or fail to recognize problems we actually had *before* the event.

If our compensation-claim fight drags on over a long time, as many will, we may, over that time, develop new problems either caused or not caused by the initial event. We may wrongly come to believe that simply because the new problem followed the initial event the new problem must have been caused by our initial event.

Our chronic problems which may, or may not, relate to our work are difficult for anyone to assess. Was our inflamed shoulder caused by our work activity or by our playing golf or is it simply part of aging or being overweight?

To make such a determination about accident- or work-related problems as accurately as possible is a complicated scientific process.

Activities of Daily Living

"Activities of Daily Living" (often written as ADL) describe the things we each need to do on a daily basis. Activities of daily living, our ability to perform these necessary activities now and in the future, ought to generally be our primary health focus. Health professionals use our ability or inability to perform activities of daily living as a measure of functional status.

Basic activities of daily living include our bathing, bladder and bowel management, care of any personal devices we may use, dressing, eating, functional mobility, personal grooming, sexual activity, sleep and rest, showering, and other similar activities.

"Instrumental" activities of daily living are not necessary for basic functioning but permit us to live independently in the community. These include our care of others, care of pets, child rearing, communication mobility, financial management, health management and maintenance, home establishment and maintenance, meal preparation and cleanup, safety procedures and emergency responses, shopping, and other similar activities.

It is important to always let our healthcare providers know about any chronic or significant problems we may be having with daily living activities. Useful forms we can print, fill in, and give to our doctors and others (so they can better understand our situations) are available at www.livingabled.com.

Maximal Medical Improvement

Whenever we are injured or ill we will always be concerned with how long our recovery will take. This may become particularly important if we are making a vehicle accident, personal injury, or workers' compensation claim. Our recovery date may either end or trigger certain compensations.

Maximal medical improvement (MMI) describes the point at which our condition has stabilized and is unlikely to get either substantially better or worse in the future. While our symptoms and signs from this condition may come and go, changes in our overall recovery or deterioration are no longer expected.

Maximal medical improvement is particularly significant in workers' compensation claims as it reflects the difference between our temporary and permanent situations. Many compensation systems define any remaining impairment or disability as "permanent" when we are determined to be at "maximal medical improvement"—which is just another way of saying we are now as good as we are likely to get.

Our time to reach maximal medical improvement may vary from days (with a minor soft-tissue injury such as a bruise or sprain) to years (if we have suffered a catastrophic injury such as significant brain trauma). While with many serious conditions our maximal medical improvement could take a year or more, appropriate therapy—along with our hard work and positive attitude—may significantly shorten this time.

Our maximal medical improvement evaluation, even when accurate, is more a comment on our bodies than on our minds or spirit. There is almost always much our minds and spirit can still do to improve our lives.

Impairment

Sam injures his arm, is treated, and a year later his doctor states that Sam has reached maximal medical improvement. Sam's doctor rates his impairment as 9 percent whole person permanent impairment based on generally accepted criteria. Sam is in constant pain and cannot return to his job as a construction laborer. Sam is confused why, when he is so disabled he can no longer work his job as a construction laborer, he has such a low impairment rating.

When injury or illness damages our ability to function, physically or mentally, temporarily or for the rest of our lives, this may be called an "impairment." *Impairment* is our loss, loss of use, or an abnormality of some part of our bodies. Our function is considered in terms of our ability to perform our activities of daily living, what we expect to do most days.

Not all conditions and diseases result in impairment. The amount of impairment depends on the severity of the condition and on us as individuals. One of us may have our broken bone heal without any permanent problems (no impairment) while another may have the same bone break and be left with decreased motion and/or a deformity.

Impairment results when our healthcare is unsuccessful in restoring our normal health. Our medical and surgical treatments are intended to support our healing and improve our function—to minimize any possible impairment. This is not always possible with such problems as amputations or brain injuries.

If we have surgery we should expect our surgery to improve our performance of our activities of daily living. Our impairment should be reduced or eliminated. Any medical treatment should leave us less impaired. The unfortunate truth, however, is that all medical treatments carry some risk and may lead to bad outcomes and greater impairment.

If our injury or illness is from an accident or is work-related our doctors are often required to determine our permanent impairment rating. Typically this is based on a book published by the American Medical Association called the *Guides to the Evaluation of Permanent Impairment* and expressed as a percentage, from 0 to 100, of loss of "whole person" function. Impairment ratings may reflect our loss or loss of use of a part of our body such as an arm, hand, leg, or foot. We would be permanently comatose or nearly dead to be assigned an impairment rating of 100 percent.

Impairment ratings are often used in workers' compensation claims to determine the amount of compensation. The more we are damaged the greater our impairment and the larger our compensation settlement.

Most doctors, unfortunately, never trained for impairment calculations. Like doing taxes, if doctors only occasionally make such calculations the process will be slow and their result likely wrong.

Some doctors calculate to show how successful they have been in restoring function. They may generate lower-than-appropriate impairment ratings. Other doctors generate higher-than-appropriate impairment ratings thinking they are helping us or more fairly representing their beliefs regarding our impairment. We, or our lawyers, may seek higher impairment ratings since these may generate more compensation.

But the goal of our healing process should be to have little or no lasting impairment. We want to fully restore or even improve our previous level of functioning. If we are told we are more impaired than we actually are, and if we work to establish that we are more impaired than we actually are, we may come to believe and actually become more impaired than we need to be.

If we face a system using impairment ratings we want to be sure the doctor calculating our rating knows how to do this accurately. If not we need to find a doctor who does. But we should never believe our impairment rating defines what we can do or that any measurement determines we face a life of disability.

Disability

Disability is a separate concept from impairment. Disability is the gap between what we can do and what we need to do.

Disability is measured as our limitation and/or restriction in certain activities. This may be determined by our failing to meet certain functional requirements or by our inability to return to our jobs. We become defined as disabled if we lack adequate ability to accomplish what we need to do.

Injury or illness may result in our not being able to accomplish certain activities, sometimes including our jobs. There is only a limited correlation between our illness or disability and our (in)capacity for work.

We define disability in terms of its timeframe and severity. Disability may be temporary or it may be permanent. It may be partial and limit only some activities or it may be total and we may be unable to perform any meaningful tasks.

Temporary partial disability (TPD) is common when we have a sudden and severe injury or illness and are temporarily unable to carry out some of our usual activities. We may have hurt our arm and not be able to use it until it heals. Permanent partial disability

(PPD) occurs when we face lifelong limitations on some activities. We have permanent loss of motion or strength in some part of our body. Permanent total disability (PTD) is associated with severe injuries or illnesses—thankfully this is not common.

The relationship between our impairment and disability is often difficult to determine. Depending on what we do for our living we may be impaired but not be disabled. A teacher may lose an arm, yet still be able to teach. Or we may have only a relatively small impairment rating yet be totally disabled for our work. If we have non-specific back pain, we may have a rating of only 3 percent or less whole person permanent impairment. If our work involves heavy lifting, we still might not be able to return to our job. It all depends. Many systems, unfortunately many workers' compensation systems, consider impairment the same as disability.

Our experience of being disabled reflects our individual perceptions and the perceptions of those interacting with us. Those of us who may be impaired are not disabled if our impairments do not stop us from performing our jobs, if we are motivated to deal with our challenges, and if others are willing to work with us to help accommodate the difficulties we face.

We want to look again at Sam, described earlier, whose arm problem resulted in a 9 percent impairment rating. As Sam was a construction laborer performing heavy lifting requiring the use of both arms he was not able to return to his job. Sam was "disabled" for working as a laborer—but not necessarily for other work. If Sam had been working a clerical job and was provided suitable accommodations, he might have faced no disability.

If our ring finger is cut off we would have an impairment rating of 100 percent for our finger (it is gone), a 10 percent impairment rating for our hand, a 9 percent impairment rating for our arm, or a 5 percent impairment rating for our whole person—there are many different ways impairment is measured.

A concert pianist would have a serious problem and probably be unable to ever again perform her profession. She might still accomplish playing the piano but probably not at the level needed for concert performances. If she were a lawyer, she would still be able to practice law and not be disabled (or only marginally disabled if she had used that finger for typing and now typed less quickly).

To assess disability we need to determine where we are actually limited or restricted. This is more complex than it may seem. Our doctors may be asked to assess our disability—but many doctors are not comfortable with disability assessments and their assessments may be inconsistent.

Doctors' recommendations regarding limiting our activities and about returning to our jobs after injury are also inconsistent. Doctors' recommendations may more reflect their beliefs regarding pain or their desire to please us than any objective reality. Doctors often respond to our requests. Our doctors may find it difficult to legitimately determine if we are disabled.

Over the years our collective beliefs about disability have been shifting. Some of us with significant physical and/or psychological limitations are now recognized as challenged but not disabled. There is also increasing recognition that even when we are disabled we have the same basic rights as those who are not. We share the right to participate in society and to lead ordinary—or extraordinary—lives. If we are disabled, however, we will face challenges to achieving our goals quite different from those faced by others. Even those of us facing significant limitations and serious disabilities retain the right to joyful and productive lives.

Disability Duration Guidelines

The premise of data-driven medicine is that, with enough data on actual patient cases, healthcare providers may rely on analysis of that data for "real-world" information. Recommendations based on data-driven medicine are specific and designed for immediate use.

One example of data-driven medicine is the collection and processing of millions of records from years of injury cases to develop disability duration guidelines. Time away from work caused by specific medical conditions was carefully analyzed. The record of average time away from work historically served as a reference for estimating how many days others with the same condition would need to return to work.

But the outcomes of past return-to-work "systems" have not been regarded by medical science as successful. "Average time away from work" has not been considered by medical scientists as an acceptable goal for avoiding needless disablement. Occupational health specialists working with statisticians looked for more complex patterns in the records to identify realistic shorter target times for return to work. These targets, also expressed in days, are based upon our expected physiological recovery from specific medical conditions. Current target times for our return to work are now often only a tenth of the earlier actual average time away from work. The new guidelines focus on our natural healing processes while considering the level of activity we need to perform a given job.

"Minimum duration" identifies the time during which the *risk* of our performing a job, to us as the injured worker or to our co-workers, is too great to return to work. This medically *required* time off work is often surprisingly short for almost all medical conditions.

"Optimum durations," corresponding to our *capacity* to work at increasingly difficult levels, follow the "minimum duration." With high-quality care and active participation from all parties, getting back to work is almost always possible during this period.

"Maximum duration" identifies the time beyond which there is almost always no longer a medical reason for disability. When cases extend beyond the "maximum duration" the question is usually one of *tolerance*–indicating we are not willing to cope with, or "tolerate," our symptoms in exchange for earning our pay. Arguably, if our pay was increased or our supervisor replaced or whatever other major concern we have with our job was changed, we might quickly decide we actually do have the capacity to return to our job.

Disability duration guidelines effectively separate the medical aspects of our recovery from the non-medical aspects. If we return to our jobs according to our natural healing, we will reap both health and productivity rewards.

i

5

What Hurts Us?

I was scared when I was told I had degenerative disc disease. This came from a doctor my lawyer had suggested. Supposedly my neck pain would never go away.
Later my primary care doctor told me the problems shown on my tests were, just like my graying hair, basically aging and not really any disease.
The more I understood the less I was scared. The less I was scared the less I hurt.

Naming Stuff

When we talk about what hurts us we want to start by identifying the problem. Once we have a problem identified, "diagnosed," we can see how concerned we need to be and think about what sort of response or treatment would be best.

As our doctors identify our problems they assign them names and these names are our diagnoses. Often these names will be in technical medical terms that may easily confuse us. If we do not completely understand what our healthcare providers are telling us, we need to immediately stop them and insist they explain things to us in terms we can understand—no matter how long that might take.

Sometimes a diagnosis may be specific, such as being told we have a "lumbar vertebral compression fracture of 20 percent"; this means we have a squished vertebra bone in our lower back. Other times a diagnosis may be descriptive, such as "non-specific low-back pain," or simply reflect symptoms, such as "arm pain." Doctors may sometimes describe

ʃ

our problems as a "syndrome," which means an association of certain characteristics which make up a problem. We may have symptoms but these may not be associated with any identifiable disease.

It is common, but wrong, for healthcare providers to use our diagnosis as a "label" to identify us as patients. This is not something that happens only in healthcare. Mechanics will identify cars as "the brake job" or "the alternator replacement" rather than as "the blue Ford." This makes little difference when talking about our cars, but a lot of difference when talking about us.

Naming us using our diagnosis, our being identified by our injury or illness label, may cause us real problems. Accepting an injury or illness label categorizes us a patient. This can lead to the loss of our freedom to make choices and decisions.

A label may be used to legitimize medical intervention and control. It sometimes also leads to our accepting the "sick role," freeing us from personal responsibilities such as our jobs.

Over time we may establish new behavior patterns based on our label. Accepting an injury or illness label may lower our chances of finding or keeping a job. An even bigger worry than what others may think of us is how we may come to think of ourselves. If we accept our diagnosis as "us," we may begin to believe our future will be our diagnosis—and that can be really bad. We may, possibly unnecessarily, become afflicted by "chronic pain."

All of us will sometimes hurt, sometimes a little and sometimes a lot, but not all pain means we have a significant injury or illness. Sometimes pain will lead doctors to identify real problems to which we should pay attention. But sometimes doctors will misinterpret what we feel and wrongly assign us a diagnosis. We need to ask doctors to explain the significance of our diagnoses.

We will generally pay a lot of attention to our diagnosis—whether it is right or wrong. If it is right, this attention can help up deal with our problem. If it is wrong, we may receive unneeded and sometimes risky treatments. The consequences of a wrong diagnosis can be serious, even deadly.

Hannah had a painful arm and was diagnosed as having "complex regional pain syndrome." She was advised that this was potentially a severe, lifelong problem. Hannah was treated with multiple medications including narcotic opioids and injections. She became addicted to the opioids and avoided using her arm. Because she stopped using it, Hannah's arm became weak.

In reality there was no evidence Hannah had ever had any problem more severe than tendinitis—which would have gotten better without treatment.

We may also have problems if medical testing reveals findings that are interpreted as "abnormal" but do not reflect a real problem.

As we get older, backbone, "spinal," degenerative-disc findings are common reports from imaging studies. Typically degenerating discs are associated with our genetics and just how long we've been living. So a study revealing these findings to us when we are middle-aged or older may not be clinically significant. However, if a doctor tells us we have degenerative disc disease, we may worry for no real reason or possibly, even worse, seek unnecessary treatment such as surgery.

Aging changes may also occur in other parts of our body. Our shoulders, for example, will likely have changes in the rotator-cuff muscles, cartilage, and tendons. Similar changes also occur in our knees and other joints. Many of these changes are simply associated with getting older. These changes may, or may not, require medical or surgical interventions.

Misleading Labels

Fatigue and pain are common reasons for visits to our doctors. Many times our doctors will not find objective physical evidence of organic injury or illness. For most of our insurance systems, our doctors are required to assign us a diagnosis before they can be paid. Sometimes, when no explainable cause is found for our complaints, our symptoms may be assigned labels for which doctors have no medical explanation. These unexplainable labels may then become us.

Humanity has always had to live with symptoms we cannot yet identify with medical testing. Medicine has yet to fully understand our bodies or our minds. But the way in which our unexplained symptoms are described and labeled has evolved throughout history and across cultures.

Common Health Conditions

Common health conditions, often pain-related disorders, can result in significant problems, including disability. Diagnoses may often be nonspecific. The assessment may be based primarily on reports of symptoms. Long-lasting and recurring low-back pain is one example.

Some doctors define some pain-related disorders as subjective health complaints or "medically unexplained symptoms." From a medical perspective these problems may be considered less severe. Those of us experiencing these problems would likely disagree. Our symptoms may cause us considerable suffering, necessitate healthcare, and result in restrictions. Many of us have symptoms that do not necessarily reflect disease. We need to identify whether our problems reflect a significant health issue or simply are part of our life.

Our understanding of the effects of these common conditions may be helped by research done in the United Kingdom. Gordon Waddell, an internationally recognized orthopedic surgeon associated with the Unum Centre for Psychosocial (relating to the interrelation of our mind and social factors) and Disability Research, Cardiff University, and Kim Burton of the Center for Health and Social Care Research, University of Huddersfield, studied disability associated with common health problems. They found no clear reason why these health problems should result in long-term incapacity, noting:

- There is usually little evidence of disease, permanent damage, or impairment.
- These conditions are common, that is, there is high background prevalence in the general (working) population.
- Many people with these conditions, even those on compensation or social-security benefits, do not have any absolute physical or mental incapacity for most ordinary activities and most jobs in modern society.
- Most sudden and severe episodes settle quite quickly (often without the need for healthcare), at least sufficiently to return to most normal activities, even if with some long-lasting or recurrent symptoms.
- Most people with these conditions remain at work and the large majority of those who do take sickness absence return to work quite quickly, even if still with some symptoms.

When our problems match these common conditions, what many of us need most is the reassurance that we can expect to recover. If our doctors recommend diagnostic studies, we want to ask why—and whether the tests or study results will change our treatment. Treatment for most of these conditions is straightforward: stay physically active and focus on what we can do and not on our symptoms. Most likely, with some time and effort, we will feel better.

Chronic Pain

Pain is a common reality. Long-lasting pain is identified as "chronic." It can significantly affect our lives and its treatment may be costly. Pain is a part of many injuries and illnesses. Sometimes pain may *be* the disease.

Pain may be described by where it is felt, how long it lasts, or what causes it. It may be from a single intense nervous-system stimulation, as simple as a stubbed toe, or from an immune-system reaction producing inflammation. Pain may be caused by genetic problems or be from nerve injuries or lesions on our central nervous system. Genetic factors may make some of us more sensitive to pain.

One of the challenges for medical responses to pain is that all pain is subjective—it is something we experience and can report to others but something others cannot measure from the outside. We may be asked to report pain on a scale of zero to ten, with zero being no pain at all and ten being the worst pain we can imagine—but the experience is personal. We sometimes show our pain without words by avoiding movement, grimacing, moaning, or protecting (guarding) parts of our bodies.

In the United States complaints of pain are the most common reason to visit doctors. Complaints of pain are a major reason for taking drugs, a major cause of our disabilities, and a key factor in our perceptions of quality of life and in our productivity.

Complaints of pain are costly to us and to our society. At the same time they are a massive income generator for healthcare providers, drug companies, and device manufacturers. Pain complaints are estimated to cost the United States up to $635 billion each year in medical treatments and lost productivity.

Chronic pain is a real medical challenge. Chronic pain is usually defined as pain that that lasts longer than six months (some say twelve months). Often it is pain we continue to feel even when doctors can identify no cause. Studies show that complaints of chronic pain vary broadly, from 12–80 percent, in different countries. The *perception* of chronic pain has cultural aspects.

Complaints of chronic pain affect an estimated 116 million American adults. This is more Americans than those affected by cancer, diabetes, and heart disease combined. Just how common these complaints are in America was shown in a 2011 Gallup poll of American adults: 31 percent complained of chronic back or neck pain, 26 percent complained of chronic knee or leg pain, and 18 percent complained of some other chronic pain. In total, 47 percent—very nearly half—of all American adults complained of at least one chronic pain.

Chronic pain is often associated with anger, anxiety, depression, distress, fear, frustration, or grief. Some studies show that, when physical causes cannot be identified, psychological and social factors may drive many of our complaints of chronic pain. This may be even more common when litigation is associated with our pain. Scientific studies indicate that the opportunity for compensation can become a dominant factor in our claims for chronic pain. Second to compensation, personality disorders have been identified as a significant risk factor.

Chronic pain affects our brain structure and function. Chronic pain may actually change the physical structure of our brains. Physical and functional changes have been shown in areas of our brains that process pain. Along with these physical and functional brain changes, chronic pain may affect how we feel pain, sometimes making us even more sensitive to pain. If we work at actively responding to our pain, we can sometimes reverse some of these changes.

Medications may be prescribed but, more often than not, medications (particularly narcotic opioids) may be associated with more risks than benefits; we will explore this issue in more detail later.

Chronic pain does not have to be a life sentence. Treatment involves reassurance and our focusing on our activities and function rather than on our pain. One of our major challenges is overcoming our fears that physical activity may be harmful or painful. Advancing carefully is often the key. Psychological support, particularly focused on changing our mindsets, may be useful. Studies have shown that, if we have chronic pain, being absorbed in activities or entertainment greatly diminishes our pain.

We have many ways to manage our pain. These can include alternative medicine, education, exercise, medication, and psychological support. Excellent online resources, including an online *ACPA Resource Guide to Chronic Pain Medications and Treatment,* are provided by the American Chronic Pain Association.

If we are involved in insurance claims or legal actions regarding pain or other symptoms, we are more likely to focus on the severity of our problem. The more we focus on our problem, the more changes occur in our brains and the more we may adopt harmful behaviors. This does not mean that if we have an insurance claim or a lawyer pursuing a legal claim for compensation our pain is not real—rather it means that an emphasized focus on our pain may reduce our focus on function. If doctors focus on our pain rather than on our function, we should consider changing doctors.

Pain Examples

A thorough discussion of the variety of physical or mental problems we may face is completely beyond the scope of *Living Abled and Healthy.* It will still be useful for us, however, to explore some common complaints. We can view back pain, whiplash, and fibromyalgia as examples of chronic pain problems.

Back Pain—Low-back pain is common. It is often a normal part of our living and aging. Backache is often identified as a back injury; however, usually it is not caused by an injury. One of the challenges we face is that our low-back pain has been "medicalized." It now provides more opportunities for treatment (as well as for profit for our doctors, other healthcare providers, and device manufacturers and drug companies).

Low-back injuries are the most frequently litigated workers' compensation claims. Spinal injuries are commonly reported vehicle-injury claims. Studies indicate that compensation will most likely be involved when minor trauma results in chronic serious low-back pain. These studies found "serious low-back pain episodes were most frequently seen arising spontaneously or with usual daily activities rather than involving trauma of any sort."

The most commonly reported types of back pain are "non-specific back pain" and "regional low-back pain." Generally these terms indicate the specific origin of our pain has not been identified. Sometimes our pain may be caused by a specific problem such as a herniated disc compressing and irritating a nerve root, resulting in pain radiating down our leg.

With most of our experiences of moderate low-back pain, our doctors' role should be to counsel and reassure us. The vast majority of time, back pain will improve on its own. All that is typically required is for us to exercise (first stretching and later strengthening) and possibly to make limited use of mild pain medications.

In today's United States (and in many other countries) this is not, unfortunately, our usual treatment. Doctors, other healthcare providers, and device manufacturers and drug companies have generated countless treatments (including injections and surgeries), gadgets, and drugs. Many of these have been scientifically demonstrated not to help—but many of us will end up trying as many of these as we can.

We need not accept this. If our healthcare providers are responding to our moderate low-back pain by immediately ordering extensive and expensive testing, developing elaborate treatment programs, or prescribing multiple medications or devices (such as back braces), we should consider whether we are seeing the appropriate providers. It is possible these providers are providing more benefits to their practices than to us.

Whiplash—"Whiplash"-associated disorder is a controversial non-medical term describing neck pain resulting from a sudden movement bending back the neck. Typically it is associated with vehicle accidents when our vehicle has been hit from behind. Popular media communicates the social acceptability of whiplash injuries.

Typically all the treatment we need is reassurance, stretching exercises, and non-prescription pain medications. Most symptoms will go away within a few days. Research indicates chronic whiplash symptoms are uncommon and most cases of whiplash resolve without permanent impairment.

Often whiplash is identified as a cause for an insurance claim or litigation. Factors influencing chronic whiplash symptoms include how badly we were hurt, pre-existing problems (physical and/or mental), expectations of pain and disability following injury, cultural influences, and mental and/or social stressors. Expectations of disability, family history, or blaming pre-existing symptoms on accidents appear to be important factors in reports of whiplash syndrome.

Some healthcare practitioners base their practices on treating vehicular injuries. They may offer us an exaggerated impression of the trauma underlying our complaints. Inaccurate diagnoses, unnecessary studies, and questionable treatments may create a false belief that we have serious problems. Lawyers may exaggerate our appropriate compensation—often we will not feel free to recover until our claim or lawsuit is settled. Or, before we know how serious our injuries may be or how long they may affect us, insurers may want to settle and close our claims. Any of these outside influences may delay our recovery.

Some doctors do not follow evidence-based guidelines and may provide us unnecessary treatment. We may be advised by such doctors to be in treatment for months. These treatments may keep us focused on pain, they may be costly, they may be risky, and they may not be the best use of our time.

We should be wary of healthcare providers who advertise or promote themselves as experts in vehicle accidents. We are probably better off to rely on our own competent primary care doctors.

If a lawyer represents us we may still want to be cautious about lawyer recommendations for medical care. Many times immediate x-rays and imaging studies, such as MRI (Magnetic Resonance Imaging) scans, are not necessary. If they are recommended we should ask why. If our treatment is not simple or is not finished within a month or two, we should question our care.

Fibromyalgia—Fibromyalgia is an example of a perplexing, controversial syndrome with many unanswered questions about its causes and its symptoms. It has been defined as a complex, chronic condition characterized by widespread non-inflammatory pain in our muscles, tendons, and/or bones; severe fatigue; and sleep disturbances. The term *fibromyalgia* is derived from three Latin words: *fibro* (fibrous, the soft tissues of the body under the skin), *my* (*myo,* muscles), and *algia* (pain). Those of us with fibromyalgia may report subjective sensations of swelling and experience multiple tender points and generalized stiffness.

This somewhat common disorder is believed to affect between three and six million people in the United States, ten times as many women as men, with most between thirty-five and sixty.

Fibromyalgia challenges contemporary medicine because doctors do not yet have a good understanding of why patients have symptoms. Current research suggests that fibromyalgia could involve imbalances in the brain and blood chemicals regulating how we perceive pain—but we have no definitive answers. There are currently no known visible clinical signs for fibromyalgia and the condition cannot yet be identified by objective laboratory tests.

Today many healthcare practitioners feel fibromyalgia is best addressed from a biopsychosocial perspective considering the relationships among our bodies, our minds, and our environment. Regardless of whether we find a clear understanding of what causes fibromyalgia and develop specific testing, proven treatment includes activity and exercise.

Some healthcare practitioners suggest that "Functional Somatic Syndrome" or "Medically Unexplained Symptoms" are more accurate descriptions of fibromyalgia and several related syndromes. Related syndromes include chronic fatigue syndrome, chronic whiplash syndrome, irritable bowel syndrome, and multiple chemical sensitivities. These syndromes are characterized by disability, suffering, and symptoms rather than by consistently demonstrable tissue abnormalities or objective diagnostic standards.

Some of us exhibiting these syndromes may offer doctors detailed self-diagnoses and find that medical explanation, reassurance, or standard symptomatic treatments provide us little relief. In some cases suffering may only be exacerbated by incorrectly attributing often-common symptoms to serious abnormalities not currently identifiable by available medical testing.

Contemporary medicine is as lacking in proven treatments for these syndromes as it is in objective clinical measurements. Typically, focusing on healthy lifestyle choices including exercise, possibly some dietary restrictions, not smoking, and weight control, rather than focusing on symptoms, will improve function and minimize difficulties.

What Do We Do?

We need to be cautious about accepting diagnostic labels. We need correct diagnoses to get correct treatment. Accepting inaccurate diagnoses may harm us by sending us down paths of extensive treatments for problems we do not have or for problems for which medicine currently can provide no proven relief. Inaccurate diagnoses and inappropriate treatments may delay us from identifying actual problems and receiving appropriate treatments. Inaccurate diagnoses may be assigned for conditions when current medicine cannot provide an adequate explanation for our experience.

We need to always inquire how diagnoses have been reached and be skeptical of those for which there is no objective foundation. Sadly, we must also always be aware that some diagnoses may be defined not for our benefit but for the benefit of others.

6

Are We or Aren't We?

Things started changing when I realized I control my
life and my health.
I had had a tough time as a kid. When I realized
how those times still affected me as an adult I began
gaining control of some of my issues.
I still have real problems. I can't deny that. Now,
though, I make better choices about my actions and,
most of all, my attitude.
My life is definitely getting better.

Beliefs

We face this question about both our health and our possible disability. Are we healthy or not? Are we disabled or not? How do we know? Why are some of us more likely to become disabled than others?

Cheryl's car is hit from behind by another car. The accident produces little damage to either car and the drivers exchange insurance information and both drive away. The next day Cheryl experiences some minor neck pain. She takes the day off to see her doctor just to make sure she has suffered no serious injury. Feeling a bit better a day later, she returns to her construction job. Cheryl's remaining neck pain gradually goes away over the following week.

Andrew is driving when his car is also rear-ended in an accident similar to Cheryl's and producing little damage. The next day he, too, experiences neck pain. He sees an injury specialist doctor the next day—and then sees a lawyer. From what the injury specialist doctor and his lawyer tell him, Andrew concludes he is going to need extensive treatment. He also concludes he won't be able to return to his job as a clerk for at least a month—maybe longer. Andrew is convinced he is experiencing severe pain and that he now has a serious problem.

Our beliefs include those we develop about our situations, particularly our expectations about our futures. Our beliefs shape how we see the world and what we perceive—even leading us to perceptions not always consistent with reality.

Our concepts of health and disability are shaped by our beliefs. If we believe our pain is severe, that it disables us, and that it is permanent, this may well become our experience. As noted in earlier discussions, our thoughts create changes in our brains and these changes affect our bodies.

Our underlying beliefs often begin in our childhoods. They are initially formed by our experiences with our families and gradually added to through our interactions with others. We will often adopt beliefs conveyed by those we see as authority figures—usually parents and other older family members, teachers, doctors, and, sometimes, lawyers. Beliefs conveyed by such authority figures will frequently become incorporated, sometimes consciously or often, especially when we are younger, unconsciously, into our own belief systems.

Our tendency will be to more likely accept new ideas consistent with our underlying beliefs and more likely reject other ideas inconsistent with our underlying beliefs. Repeated exposure to assertions—even those for which we have no evidence—increases our likelihood to believe these assertions.

Our beliefs about any injury or illness we may experience will shape how both we and our doctors respond to our problem. Recognizing and understanding underlying beliefs can help us better understand and even change our subjective experience, improve our capacity to cope, increase the effectiveness of our treatment, and speed recovery.

Our perceptions of injury or illness often offer a better prediction of our recovery than objective measurements taken by our doctors. When we are more positive about our future we are more likely to have better functional outcomes.

Locus of Control

Jim complains "Why does this always happen to me? My doctor is supposed to be fixing me and she isn't. My lawyer hasn't contacted me for months and I want him to get me the money I deserve."

Cathy always "takes the bull by the horns." She exerts herself and she is in control of her life. She assumes responsibility for her actions.

Jim and Cathy experience life differently. Jim complains about others while Cathy takes control.

Our success in life may be strongly affected by our beliefs in whether or not we control our lives and our future. "Locus of control" describes our expectations concerning whether or not we control events in our lives.

Seeing Strengths

When he was just two years old Craig MacFarlane blinded his left eye while playing with an igniter for welding torches. Six weeks later his right eye went blind in a "sympathetic response" to the loss of vision in the injured eye. By the time he was two-and-a-half Craig MacFarlane was completely blind.

His parents, however, never allowed his blindness to be a limiting handicap. He was always included in their family camping, fishing, and hiking activities.

At six, MacFarlane started attending a school for the blind. There he began competitive wrestling and went on to win numerous medals. He learned the clarinet, piano, trombone, and trumpet. Later he became active in numerous other sports, including track and skiing, with great accomplishment.

Howard Cosell reported "I've covered the sports beat for nearly forty years of my life and worked with all the great ones firsthand. Jackie Roosevelt Robinson, Muhammad Ali, Johnny McEnroe... you name them. But I must tell you the most remarkable athlete I have ever seen—ever known—is Craig MacFarlane."

MacFarlane's message is to not consider our limitations as handicaps; they may become our uniqueness and strengths. MacFarlane considers his blindness just a "minor inconvenience" rather than a handicap.

If we see ourselves as mostly in control of our lives we have an "internal" locus of control. If we see ourselves as mostly *not* in control, but subject more to chance or others' control, we have an "external" locus of control. The question we need to ask is, "Who is in control of my life?"

Our having an internal locus of control is empowering—but it can also be frightening to acknowledge our own control. In our lives all of us make mistakes and there are consequences. Our having an external locus of control may be a psychological defense—if we are not in control then things just happen to us and we are not responsible. It was someone else's fault.

If we face health issues we may wish and wait for others to "make us better." If this is our focus, we may feel less need to recognize our personal responsibility. But the reality is that, while we will face situations we did nothing to create, we each play the central role in what happens in our lives and how we choose to live our lives. If we see ourselves as helpless, then we will be helpless. But if, even if we face catastrophic events, we always recognize our strengths and our personal responsibility for our futures, we will do better. We can make our lives more difficult by completely turning control of our medical issues over to our doctors. Their advice is important, but we must take responsibility and educate ourselves about what our doctors recommend—particularly when it comes to invasive procedures and surgeries.

Am I at Risk?

Emily has had a tough life. As a child she was physically abused and as a teenager she was raped. She does not share any of that past. Her past still haunts her. Emily feels the world is still out to get her. She takes comfort in food, does not like to exercise, and smokes cigarettes. Emily is depressed, hates her job, and is a loner.

Kim experienced a happy childhood and was nurtured by loving parents. She embraces life, exercises, and eats wisely. Kim approaches each day with a positive attitude.

What makes us more likely to not recover from serious health problems? What do *we* do that may lead to our disability? When we recognize what puts us at greater risk we can take action to lessen that risk.

Much scientific research has focused on what predicts whether or not we are likely to face a "delayed recovery"—taking longer to recover than would be expected for our health problems. How we think about our health problems helps determine how these problems affect us. Issues relating to our speed of recovery include:

- Attitude—Are we positive or negative?
- Beliefs—What do we believe about our recovery?
- Locus of Control—Where do we see control located, is it internal or external? Are we in control or are others in control?
- Coping Skills—How do we deal with stress and other challenges?
- Resiliency—How resilient are we in dealing with life's challenges?
- Health—How healthy, in body, mind, and spirit, did we keep ourselves *before* our current problem?

If we cannot successfully recognize our control and responsibility in these factors we are more likely to allow our symptoms to control our lives.

Research has focused on identifying "risk factors" relating to our speed of recovery from health problems. We should recognize how these risk factors affect both us and those we care about.

- Physical issues—Are we older? Is our problem more or less serious? Were we healthy and in good condition before our current problem? Are we overweight? Do we smoke? Do we abuse alcohol and/or other drugs?
- Behavior—Were we abused when we were children? Has it taken us longer than expected to recover from prior health problems? Do we have difficulties coping? Do we have a history of insurance claims or litigation?
- Personality disorders—Do we have trouble perceiving and relating to situations and to people? Do we have rigid and unhealthy patterns of thinking and behaving interfering with our experiencing joyful and productive lives?
- Psychological—Do we have anxiety, depression, or other psychological issues? Are we angry?
- Healthcare—Have we been accurately informed about our conditions and has the healthcare proposed for us or provided to us been appropriate?
- Psychosocial—Do we lack support? Does our home and personal life support our recovery? Do we want revenge?

- Litigation—Have we involved lawyers and have we controlled their priorities?
- Cultural—What are our cultural expectations regarding our health issues?
- Work—Do we like our jobs, supervisors, and co-workers? Do we receive positive feedback in our jobs? Do we have control over our jobs? Does our employer provide programs supporting our gradual return to our jobs and welcome us back to our jobs?

How do our expectations about disability relate to our jobs? Studies show that beliefs that our health problems are work-based lead to poorer outcomes. This often is the result of the challenges we face with our compensation and legal systems and the negative affects we face from hearings or litigation. If we have low expectations and believe we do not have the physical and/or mental capacity to return to our jobs, we will be less likely to successfully return.

We are more likely to quickly return to work when we have earlier developed coping skills, health literacy, a positive attitude, and resiliency. This is enhanced if we respect our employer and recognize cultural or moral obligations to our job commitments. Our perceptions of health and our jobs profoundly affect whether or not we allow ourselves to become disabled.

When we enjoy our jobs, feel supported by coworkers and employers, and believe our jobs benefit others we are more likely to quickly return to them. A health problem, even one that may be substantial and/or long lasting, does not have to mean we are disabled and cannot return to work.

Childhoods and Early Life Experiences

Childhoods play major roles in shaping who we become as adults. A childhood history of problems dealing with others and difficulties setting and achieving goals may often predict future problems in our adult lives and jobs.

Upsetting early life experiences (especially physical, mental, or sexual abuse), less-than-adequate parenting, and a lack of positive guidance in our childhoods and adolescence may hurt us then and later in life. We, personally, and our larger society may pay a price in our increased health, disability, and social services costs; in our higher probability of becoming involved with the criminal justice system; and simply in our greater likelihood of personal unhappiness.

Science continues to develop better understandings of the relationship between our childhood events and our health later in life. The "Adverse Childhood Experiences" study is a collaborative research effort involving the U.S. Centers for Disease Control and Prevention (based in Atlanta, Georgia) and Kaiser Permanente's Health Appraisal Clinic (in San Diego, California). Between 1995 and 1997 over seventeen thousand Kaiser Permanente members voluntarily completed a survey identifying harsh events in their childhoods as well as their then-current health status. Researchers continue tracking the medical status of these baseline participants to better understand how stressful or traumatic experiences in our childhood affect our adult health.

Of the study participants reporting adverse childhood experiences
- 28 percent experienced physical abuse;
- 27 percent grew up with someone in their household abusing alcohol and/or other drugs;
- 23 percent lost a parent to separation or divorce;
- 21 percent experienced sexual abuse;
- 19 percent grew up with a mentally ill person in their household;
- 15 percent experienced emotional neglect;
- 13 percent witnessed their mothers being treated violently;
- 11 percent experienced emotional abuse;
- 10 percent experienced physical neglect;
- 5 percent grew up with a household member in jail or prison.

As the Centers for Disease Control and Prevention processed the study participants' information they found that 63 percent of the participants had endured at least one study category of childhood trauma and that over 20 percent of the participants had endured three or more. Probably most of us have encountered some childhood trauma.

Childhood adversity correlated with development of depression, post-traumatic stress disorders, and suicide attempts. Childhood adversity also correlated with a greater likelihood of poor health behaviors such as alcohol and/or other drug abuse, obesity, smoking, and, generally, a poor health-related quality of life. Adverse childhood experiences also increased our risk of medical problems including chronic obstructive pulmonary disease, ischemic heart disease, and liver disease.

The study assessed the relationship between eight types of adverse childhood experiences and our serious job problems, financial problems, and work absenteeism and found strong evidence of a relationship between our adverse childhood experiences and poor performance at our jobs. Long-term effects of adverse childhood experiences on the workforce as a whole were concluded to impose preventable major human and economic costs.

When we are looking deeply into what current aspects of our lives may be driving some of our negative behaviors we ought to also be looking at:

- Were we physically abused as a child?
- Were we sexually molested as a child or adolescent?
- Have we ever been raped?
- Has anyone in our family been murdered?
- Has anyone in our family had a nervous breakdown?
- Has anyone in our family committed suicide?
- Has anyone in our family abused alcohol and/or other drugs?
- Have we ever been in combat?
- Have we ever lived in a war zone?

Do any of these risk factors apply to us? Recognizing these risk factors should encourage us to seek assistance in dealing with our issues. If we are experiencing chronic pain or disability and have any of these risk factors, we should share this information with our doctors.

Confronting Challenges

Victor Marx faced horrendous abuse as a child. His absentee father was a pimp and a drug dealer. At five Marx was sexually molested and left for dead in a cooler. As a teenager he endured abuse from several stepfathers and attended fourteen different schools. He tried to escape his emotional pain with drugs; that didn't work.

As an adult he was diagnosed with mental illness and post-traumatic stress disorder (PTSD). He sought counseling and confronted his challenges. He made the choice to be victorious rather than stay a victim.

He also developed his skills—including earning a seventh-degree black belt in what he identifies as "Cajun Karate Keichu-do" (a mixture of karate, jui-jitsu, and boxing). Marx is now president of "All Things Possible," a national faith-based organization. He travels the globe delivering a message of hope and restoration focusing on the needs of troubled and hurting youth. His wife works side by side with him, sharing his passion to prevent abuse and empower those with troubled pasts.

Many of us facing Marx's challenges would not have been as victorious. We likely would have attempted to suppress our past and would still experience flashbacks of the horrors we endured. We would probably still experience pain (emotional and physical) and perpetuate the abuse cycle with our spouses and children. Continued drug abuse and other illegal activities would be common responses. By recognizing, acknowledging, and successfully confronting his past, Marx chose a different life.

A history of adverse childhood experiences does not condemn us to problems as adults. It should, however, alert us to our possible risk for delayed recovery and/or poor outcomes from treatments. A history of adverse childhood experiences does not excuse us from responsibility for our own current actions.

Personality Disorders

Our personalities are unique and may sometimes be challenging. The human psyche—the totality of the human brain, conscious and unconscious thought—is complex.

We all know people we would describe as "unusual" or who behave oddly. Sometimes we are these people. Some of us may have what is known as "personality disorders." If we do have a personality disorder, it is something for us to recognize and address. Avoiding and not acknowledging our issues will only continue to harm us.

Personality disorders are recognized by our enduring patterns of inner experience and behaviors deviating markedly from those expected by our culture. These patterns are pervasive and inflexible and often begin in our adolescence or early adulthood. Personality disorders are relatively stable over time and can lead to distress or impairment. Often we may just have distinctive personality traits as opposed to disorders. The defining difference will be that our distinctive personality traits will not seriously affect our ability to function in our activities of daily living—both basic and instrumental.

Symptoms currently defined as personality disorders in contemporary American society are common. They are seen in 10–15 percent of the general U.S. population.

There are different types of personality disorders. Movies offer us some examples—typically extreme examples rarely matched in everyday life. Most often our personality disorders, or personality traits, are vastly subtler.

In *Fatal Attraction,* a 1987 thriller, Michael Douglas plays a New York lawyer stalked by a woman, played by Glenn Close, with whom he has had an affair. The woman stalker, who has a borderline personality disorder, demonstrates patterns of instability in interpersonal relationships and self-image and a lack of impulse control.

Gone With the Wind is a 1939 romantic epic set during the American Civil War. It portrays the story of a woman manifesting histrionic personality disorder—a pattern of excessive emotionality and attention seeking.

While both of these are clearly examples of personality disorders, most of the personality disorders we may suffer are, thankfully, rarely anywhere as violent or as obvious as those shown in the movies.

What may be considered a symptom of a disorder by one culture may be perfectly acceptable to another. What is considered outside of cultural expectations also changes over time—behaviors once considered normal might now be considered a sign of a disorder.

Personality disorders generally originate early in our lives, before adulthood. Long-lasting and rigid patterns of thought and behavior may challenge our feelings, impulse control, personal relationships, and thinking.

What current medical standards recognize as personality disorders are common in today's American society. Mostly, however, neither we nor our primary care doctors will recognize the less extreme of these behaviors. Mental health specialists, usually psychologists or psychiatrists, will more commonly make these kinds of diagnoses.

We must be aware, however, that these diagnoses will not always be accurate. And, like other healthcare specialists, psychologists and psychiatrists tend to assign us "labels" and then often identify us as our "label."

In contemporary American society we will often resist being labeled with a mental or behavioral diagnosis. While most of us may accept our physical diagnoses, we frequently view a psychological diagnosis with shame. Yet personality disorders, particularly when not recognized and addressed, may profoundly affect our health and whether or not we become disabled. Personality disorders are, by their very nature, often unrecognized by those of us who have them. This is all the more reason we should stay open to assessments from trusted observers—professional and non-professional alike—and recognize our responsibility to address any issues we may face.

These long-lasting and rigid patterns of thought and behavior are more common among those of us with chronic pain. Studies indicate that many of us with chronic pain have, at least to some degree, some form of a personality disorder. We must stay open to recognizing and addressing the role our personalities play in our pain experience. What is important is for us to recognize when we or others are acting outside of currently accepted cultural norms. With that recognition we should be seeking professional assistance to help us or others address these issues.

Some disorders may be the result of childhood abuse or neglect— but that still leaves us with our personal responsibility to successfully deal with whatever problems we may now be facing. Ongoing research suggests that some personality disorders may involve genetic and/or physical factors.

The bad news about our personality disorders is that they are resistant to change. This can be frustrating both for us and for our care providers.

The good news about our personality disorders is that our treatment begins with our first recognizing and then addressing our problem through education and individual, family, or group counseling, sometimes aided by medication. It need not be frightening or overwhelming to face up to our personality issues.

While we may not completely change our underlying patterns, with time and effort we can often find ways to overcome many of our symptoms and regain greater functionality and success in maintaining our activities of daily living. If we do face such problems, we should be comforted that we are not alone. Many of us must deal with these issues—and we have many opportunities to seek help.

Dependence and Codependence

Many of us having dependency issues come from dysfunctional families. The truth is that such families are common. Psychological dependency is our preoccupation with and an extreme emotional, social, and/or physical dependence on a person or object. It is generally a reflection of having underdeveloped self-esteem combined with our inappropriate caring for another and our inappropriate reliance on this other's responses.

Dependency may also arise when we have a partner who is self-absorbed or uninterested and we become obsessive about pleasing or interesting our partner. Dependency may occur in any type of relationship—community, family, peer, romantic, work, etc. Dependency may also occur in relationships with professionals such as our counselors, doctors, or lawyers.

If our dependency comes to affect and be returned and reciprocated by the person on whom we are dependent, our relationship has then become "codependent." The concept of codependence was first formally recognized about forty years ago. Initially this concept was used to describe spouses of alcoholics—specifically those of us who stayed for long times in such relationships. Today the concept is used to describe a much broader range of relationships. Codependence often reflects a shared, exaggerated, dependent pattern of learned behaviors, beliefs, and feelings.

In either dependency or codependency we may continue in destructive and disabling relationships. Do we have relationships in our lives that might be defined as "dependent" or "codependent"? Have we perhaps developed such a relationship with our counselors, doctors, or lawyers? Can we see how moving away from such dependency or codependency would restore our independence, increase our personal freedom, and improve our lives?

Victimization

Do we blame others for our problems or do we recognize our responsibilities and shortcomings and move on with our lives? A proliferation of lawyers and lawsuits has helped push American life increasingly toward victimization and away from earlier American ideals of personal responsibility and self-reliance. Many of America's lawyers make their livings by helping to define us as victims.

What happens when we repeatedly tell ourselves and others: "I am not responsible. It's not my fault. There was nothing I could do. I am not in control"?

We may overlook the destruction these beliefs bring to our lives—we throw away our potential. Victimization will not, in the long run, benefit *us*—those who may benefit financially will be our healthcare providers and our lawyers.

Drug company advertisements would lead us to believe that all aches and pains; anxious, depressed, or distressed feelings; or our sleeping difficulties are not normal parts of our lives. If we embrace these symptoms, we are disease victims. Drug companies continually encourage us to see our doctors or psychologists to be prescribed and take their drugs and begin ongoing treatment.

We are encouraged to believe our medical care will always be passive—for every problem there is a magic drug or treatment. We are constantly being encouraged to become victims. We cannot allow ourselves to be captured in this downward spiral of victimization.

Sick Role and Illness Behavior

The concept of the "sick role" describes how contemporary American society supports the belief that those of us who are sick should not be held responsible for our illness—we should be cared for and excused from our normal obligations until we are well. Originally referring to sudden and severe illness, "sick role" is now applied as well to our chronic illnesses and disabilities.

When we come to believe our condition is unlikely to improve and accept our condition and resulting dependency as permanent our "sick role" may expand into a "disabled role." We may be using magnified physical complaints to influence others. We may be totally unaware of the reasons behind our actions.

The sick role may provide us one way to receive attention. We get to feel unique and important and may now able to exert some degree of power over others. Our sick role may be reinforced by not having to work, staying home, reduced personal responsibilities, and hopes of financial compensation.

Illness behaviors are reinforced when the behaviors increase the attention we receive from doctors, freedom to access medications, and freedom to avoid work while still receiving compensation. But these actions also serve to reduce our independence and limit our self-reliance and our ability to live empowered lives.

Somatization

We may experience somatic (body) symptoms (sensations) and have significant distress and disruption of our lives. We may perceive these symptoms as harmful, threatening, or troublesome. For some of us health concerns may become our central thoughts and we may focus time and energy everyday on health concerns.

Since physical symptoms allow us to indicate physical distress, rather than psychological distress, they justify our efforts to seek medical attention. For this perceived benefit, between 5 and 7 percent of us may, consciously or unconsciously, generate physical symptoms having no identifiable physical basis.

Such symptoms *could* be the result of organic disease. This is why we, consciously or unconsciously, chose symptoms recognizable as evidence of physical disease. Doctors find no currently identifiable significant objective signs explaining presenting symptoms in 25–50 percent of primary care encounters. Specialty- or pain-clinic presentations lacking currently identifiable significant objective signs approach 60 percent.

This does not mean the symptoms we experience are not real to us. Our symptoms may or may not be associated with other medical conditions. Lacking currently identifiable objective signs may also reflect the inability of doctors to identify a physical problem or their lack of an adequate explanation for our experiences.

Western healthcare systems legitimize physical disease but not psychological disorders. They express this bias by more readily compensating our physical diseases while often reducing or denying compensation for psychological needs.

Genetic and biological vulnerability, traumatic episodes in our early lives, and learned behaviors (receiving supportive attention when ill) may all contribute to somatic symptoms. We may wrongly blame somatic symptoms on physical disease.

Some doctors may—out of an attempt at kindness, out of ignorance, out of ego, or out of their desire for personal gain—provide unprovable medical diagnoses for somatic symptoms. Unprovable diagnoses feed convictions of injury or illness and disability and may promote treatments at best benign and at worst dangerous.

When we are worried and consult multiple doctors for the same problems and are repeatedly told everything is OK, we really should consider the possibility our problems are more with our minds than our bodies. Between 1.3 and 10 percent of us have problems with illness anxiety.

When creation of these symptoms has been unconscious, as it most often is, we are truly expressing our experience. We are not consciously manipulating or controlling others through our symptoms—but manipulation or control may be occurring.

Medicalization

Medicalization is the process by which our conditions and problems come to be defined and treated as medical conditions. Alcoholism, childhood hyperactivity, obesity, sexual dysfunction, and sleep problems have all been defined as medical problems to be treated by our doctors.

When our complaints are subject to medical study, diagnosis, and treatment we may benefit by gaining a greater understanding of these conditions and, sometimes, effective therapies. Medicalization always reflects current societal views and is dependent on the prevailing concepts of health and illness.

Labeling an experience as a medical condition permits our healthcare providers to charge to treat us and provides our drug companies new markets. Why would we want to encourage them to profit at our expense?

Secondary Gain

We need to understand the dangers of a possible focus on "secondary gain." When continuing our symptoms allows us to avoid what we dislike or allows us to gain something we do like we are dealing with "secondary gain."

Brandon's back pain means he cannot work. He is getting workers' compensation and the amount is close to what he was earning before. He did not like his job and now gets to be home. His wife is more attentive than ever.

There are many types of secondary gain. We portray ourselves as unable to function and we may be cared for by those who love us. We may not have to work. We may have a convenient excuse for our behavior.

We need to look deep inside ourselves—not just superficially—and ask ourselves if we believe we are gaining some value from continuing our health problem. Then we need to assess whether it is truly to our long-term benefit, as individuals seeking our best possible lives, for us to continue our problems. Again, careful scientific studies have shown how our thoughts and the thoughts and actions of those around us may be more significant to the speed and the extent of our recoveries than actual medical issues.

Malingering

Malingering is falsely representing (feigning) injury or illness to avoid obligations or work. If we fake injury or illness or pretend to have more extreme symptoms than we really do to avoid responsibilities, we are malingering. Malingering has been reported at least since biblical times. As a boy, David, fearful of his king's wrath, "feigned himself mad."

Malingering may occur when we want to avoid prosecution or punishment, undesirable duties, work, or to obtain compensation or drugs. Malingering may be suspected if we display some of the following: a "medicolegal context of presentation" (such as if we have been referred to our doctor by a lawyer or if we reference our physical complaints to legal responsibilities); a marked discrepancy between our claimed stress or disability and our objective medical signs; a lack of cooperation during our diagnostic evaluation or in following our prescribed treatment regimen; or symptoms of antisocial personality disorder.

Malingering is a serious issue. It reflects our cultural integrity—or our lack of it.

Fraud

Fraud occurs when we or others knowingly lie to obtain benefits or advantages to which we or they are not otherwise entitled. It is also fraud if someone else knowingly denies us or others benefits to which we or they are entitled.

The usual elements of fraud are intentional deception, achieving personal gain (typically financial compensation or, often in healthcare fraud, drugs), or damage or expense to another. Fraud ranges from subtle to outright blatant.

It is difficult to know how much healthcare fraud exists since it often goes undetected. Various government authorities have estimated healthcare fraud, of both private and public providers, to be 3–10 percent of total U.S. healthcare costs.

Identified risk factors for fraud include:

- Incentive/Pressure—typically a financial need.
- Rationalization—excuses such as "They have lots of money" or "They should pay."
- Opportunity—a perceived possibility of successfully committing fraud. Often fraud begins with small amounts of money and then increases.

Most who commit fraud are not career criminals and often have no criminal history. However, with the billions of dollars involved, healthcare and disability fraud is also actively practiced by organized crime.

Governments and private insurers paying fraudulent claims ultimately end up charging us, as taxpayers and customers, to cover these costs. Why would we tolerate fraud?

What Do We Do?

Our fundamental choice is accepting our personal responsibilities or allowing others to take control of our lives. If we accept our responsibilities, we claim our freedoms and independence. We maintain control of our destiny.

We can choose to recognize the impact of our personalities, behaviors, and psychological issues. We act with integrity. While others may try to help us or harm us, in the end our lives are controlled by our choices. The challenges we face are not barriers; they are a normal part of most lives.

7

Systems and Non-Systems

*Dealing with workers' compensation was just so
confusing. Sometimes I wished I'd never even filed my
claim.*
*After getting more information and now better
understanding the process, I feel I am in better control
of what is happening.*

In the United States, when we are injured or ill, we will commonly end
up becoming involved with various so-called "systems," often including
healthcare, insurance, legal, and disability. Most of these are really not
systematic at all. The U.S. array of private and public "systems" cannot
help but confuse the best of us—often including our doctors.

Many of us will become disabled before we retire. Just over one-
in-four of twenty-years-olds will become disabled by the time they
retire. In 2010, 12 percent of the total U.S. population was classified as
disabled and more than half of these were between eighteen and sixty-
four—prime working years.

As long ago as 1870 the German Chancellor Otto von Bismarck
established what has been termed the "welfare monarchy." At that time
injured German workers were financially cared for by their government
until they returned to full health.

A limited vestige of this tradition is continued in the United States
through compensation systems including workers' compensation
systems, healthcare insurance, private disability insurance, and state-
funded and federal programs including those controlled by the U.S.

Social Security Administration, the military, and the U.S. Department of Veterans Affairs.

Depending on how and where our problem occurred, and to which compensation systems we may or may not be entitled, we will often become involved with one or more of these so-called systems. We need to be aware of our responsibilities and those of our employers and insurers.

If our medical problem cannot be associated with a specific injury and we have healthcare insurance, our healthcare insurance may provide treatment. If we do not have healthcare insurance, we may be covered by one or more state or federal programs. If we had a job but now are unable to work, we may receive short- or long-term compensation from our disability insurance. If we do not have disability insurance, we may receive compensation from our state. We may qualify for federal Social Security Disability coverage.

If our problem was caused by a work-related injury, our workers' compensation coverage may take care of medical and disability needs. We may also be provided with vocational rehabilitation. If our problem resulted from a vehicle accident, either our or someone else's vehicle insurance may take care of our medical and disability needs. If the problem resulted from someone else's negligence, they or their insurer may accept responsibility. If we are serving in the military, we may have medical coverage provided by the military or, later, by the U.S. Department of Veterans Affairs.

Because we have so many possible participants in the United States healthcare non-systems, every statement about healthcare coverage must include the word "may." We never know for sure what "will" happen to us until we face a particular problem.

Many other countries use what are called "single-payer" healthcare systems where all of those covered by the national system see their healthcare guaranteed by their governments. This is, obviously, far less confusing for those seeking healthcare and those covered are far more certain of securing their needed healthcare.

As many of us have already learned, with so many different participants in our U.S. "system," there is often a tendency for any one participant to try to shift responsibility for our problem to a different participant. If we suffer from back pain we believe was created by or in our workplace, our workers' compensation insurer or employer may or may not accept our belief that our back pain is actually work-related. If we do not have healthcare insurance coverage, we may see it to our advantage to have this filed under workers' compensation. Our employers may try to shift responsibility for our injury care to our healthcare insurer or to a government program such as Social Security. Our healthcare insurer may want to shift responsibility to the workers' compensation insurer or another responsible party. If we go to see a government program, that program may refuse us help.

It is not surprising many of us will end up confused or frustrated or both. The time we lose to this confusion may be critical to the success or failure of our healthcare. We need at least a basic understanding of these non-systems if we are to have any hope for securing our needed healthcare—especially securing it in a timely manner.

Workers' Compensation

Workers' compensation is designed to provide medical care and compensation for those of us who work and who are injured at or through our jobs. The common language defining injury or illness covered by workers' compensation is that our injury or illness "arose of and in the course of [our] employment."

Workers' compensation was historically the first social insurance program adopted by what are commonly referred to as "developed" countries. In the United States each state regulates its own workers' compensation program. There are also a variety of federal programs each servicing specific groups of workers.

In most states employers are required to publicly post information about workers' compensation. Typically what is provided is the agency, department, or person to contact.

What should we do if we believe we have been hurt at work or that our medical problem is work-related? First we must report our injury to our employer and seek appropriate care. We want to get information on how our particular workers' compensation system works. Often we can start by searching the Internet using "our state + workers' compensation" as our search term and focusing on sites we find ending in ".gov." These

".gov" sites will be our official government sites. Or we may be able to get printed information through our state's department of labor.

A list of state workers' compensation officials is provided by the U.S. Department of Labor; this link is provided in the Internet resources in the back of *Living Abled and Healthy* and is available at www.livingabled.com. We can also search Internet sites devoted to workers' compensation information such as www.workcompcentral.com and www.workerscompensation.com. We need to learn as much as we can to make wise choices and maintain control of our health.

Robert Aurbach, JD, an internationally recognized legal expert on workers' compensation, offers the following guidance:

> The first thing to understand about workers' compensation is what it is and what it is not. It is a statutory program. Our state (or, in some instances, our federal) legislative process, rather than any person or company, has determined the amount of compensation and the conditions for our eligibility for compensation. Workers' compensation is intended to create conditions where we have the opportunity to heal after our workplace injury (or illness) so that we may return to our jobs as soon as we are safely able.
>
> Workers' compensation is not designed to fully compensate us for our injuries. The majority of workers' compensation programs in the United States pay two-thirds of the average income as the maximum benefit (where two-thirds of our average income roughly approximates net pay after taxes and other deductions). Workers' compensation does not compensate us for pain and suffering, inconvenience, or loss of enjoyment of the things we used to do.
>
> Workers' compensation is designed to pay necessary medical bills with no cost to us and provide us compensation to pay other expenses while we heal. Compensation stops when we are able to go back to our jobs. Workers' compensation also attempts to compensate us for some of the income we may lose in our future from our lost future earning power if our injury is sufficiently severe. Workers' compensation is not designed to be a substitute for our returning to work. Research has shown that no U.S. system pays enough workers' compensation to equal the income we would make over the rest of our working life.

Some of us may think this system is "unfair" and that we ought to be able to get "more." Unlike compensation for other kinds of personal injury, workers' compensation was established to provide us with temporary care and support regardless of who caused the accident. It was also established under governmental control so that our employers are required to be financially responsible (usually by buying insurance) for any injuries we may incur. The medical compensation will be paid in full and we will have no co-pay for our medical expenses. The extent of this compensation, which is not matched in normal personal-injury cases, is seen by our legislatures to offset and justify our reduced level of compensation.

But the basic reality remains: None of us on workers' compensation will ever receive as much as we would have made if we were able to return to our jobs. Recognizing this reality, it is important for us to think about our best long-term interests. Research shows that the longer we stay away from our jobs the less likely we are to ever return to our jobs.

When we are injured (or even before), we should be thinking about what we want our lives to be like in our future. We want to talk about our hopes with those people who are important in our lives. Some of us may benefit from writing down our thoughts and keeping these written recordings somewhere we can always look at them.

Our decisions about what we want our lives to be can be helpful in weighing any advice we are given. Our shared and/or recorded thoughts can help us ask the right questions of those professionals treating us and representing us. If the advice we are given (from whatever source) advances our long-term goals, it is probably good advice. If the advice we are given conflicts with our long-term goals, we probably should get a second, or, sometimes, even a third, opinion before we reach our own conclusions.

Finally, if it is reasonably possible for us to do so, we want to avoid disputes. Television dramas give us the impression that going to a hearing or court is easy and everything is settled in an hour, less the commercial breaks. The reality is that going to contested case hearings or court are long, difficult, and intensely stressful processes which often take on lives of their own. We will likely be away from our jobs for an extended time. Personal relationships will often become painfully stressed. We will almost certainly feel we have lost control of the process—because, in most cases, we will have—and become frustrated with the months or years it takes for us to achieve a final resolution. At the end of the process we probably will not even go to a hearing or court because our lawyers will settle, rather than take to hearings or trials, most cases.

If we do face a dispute we want to consider all possible ways to resolve our dispute in the fastest and least-formal way possible to best preserve our true long-term interests.

Most work-related injuries involve muscles, tendons, and/or bones—frequently in the back, neck, shoulders, arms, or legs. If we suffer a sudden and severe injury at our workplace—such as tripping over something, falling, and breaking an arm—it will often be clear we are covered by workers' compensation. It may be less clear when we are suffering from a chronic condition such as pain.

With chronic conditions we can expect insurers and employers demanding to analyze all possible causes, work related and otherwise, for the problem before possibly accepting responsibility. If the problem is work-related, then they are responsible for all reasonable, appropriate, and necessary healthcare needed to address the condition.

If we become unable to work from either a sudden and severe or a chronic work-related condition, our insurer or employer must provide us disability compensation. If we suffer permanent loss of function, we should also receive compensation for permanent impairment and/or disability. In addition, some states will require we be provided with vocational rehabilitation.

The original plan for our workers' compensation system was well-intended. Unfortunately the mixed incentives now at the core of this system may end up confusing us and result in needless costs and less-healthy outcomes.

Workers' compensation coverage requires us to demonstrate that our problem occurred in our workplace or resulted from work activities for us to receive medical coverage and/or other compensation. Repeatedly demonstrating that our problem resulted from work activities requires us to maintain a negative focus on our problem. Yet we know we are more likely to have a better health outcome when we maintain a positive focus. We know that accepting responsibility for our health is healthier for us than blaming others or relying on others to "make us well."

Workers' compensation coverage contains a built-in conflict between the negative focus we need to maintain to secure the medical coverage and compensation to which the law tells us we are entitled and the positive focus we need to maintain to secure our fastest healing and best-possible health outcome.

Workers' compensation is a complex system with multiple stakeholders each having their own agenda. The incentives for some stakeholders in this system are simply not beneficial for our best interests as injured workers. Workers' compensation does not really provide incentives for our most positive health outcomes following our best-quality healthcare.

Instead workers' compensation provides more reimbursement for frequently expensive, often unnecessary, and potentially harmful medical procedures. This "system" may actually discourage doctors from educating us on what might be our best medical answers. Drugs and devices profitable for the drug and device suppliers (and our doctors) may be prescribed for us. These drugs and devices may provide questionable, if any, benefits and may even be harmful. The workers' compensation system encourages doctors to generate diagnoses (sometimes for symptoms of everyday lives) and attribute them (sometimes erroneously) to our work.

Most (although certainly not all) work-related problems, if treated appropriately, should end with recovery—leaving no permanent impairment. Yet the workers' compensation system provides greater incentives for us to be permanently impaired than it does for us to be fully recovered. As injured workers we receive larger awards when we can convince hearing officers, other decision makers, or judges we are significantly impaired and unable to return to work. The worse we can portray our problem and the greater evidence of impairment or disability we can demonstrate, the greater the compensation will be for our claim.

As the estimates of our impairment (medical estimates of loss of function) or disability become more significant the greater the probability we may involve lawyers. Our employers and/or their insurers may be represented by lawyers arguing against us—and we know how much advantage their specialized training provides them and how intimidating they can be to face without some equal representation supporting us.

When we have involved lawyers—often feeling we had no other choice—some lawyers in some states will take our cases knowing the more impaired and disabled they can prove us to be the more money they will make. In other states workers' compensation lawyers are paid by the hour—but even in such states cases involving more serious claims will generally take more time to negotiate, settle, or reach judgment. Since the possible financial rewards are now greater there is now more need for other experts, many of whom make their livings by successfully proving their clients—us—are impaired and disabled. This then becomes our reality—but not a good reality.

Some employers will ignore our well-documented health benefits from working and, if we have been injured, refuse to allow us to return to our jobs even when we are medically able to come back. Employers may use workers' compensation settlements to get rid of workers they may evaluate as "problematic" (sometimes just because we have been injured but other times because of performance issues or personality conflicts). Some employers are concerned that having a history of work-related injuries will cause their insurers to charge them larger premiums—which is exactly what does happen.

Most insurance claims adjusters want to "close" (pay any existing obligation and end any potential future liability) compensation claims as quickly as possible. Ideally closing our compensation claim will include our being covered for our appropriate treatment, restoration of full function, and returning to our jobs. Often, however, this may not be the case.

We may have issues associated with our cases resolved in hearings or with formal litigation. This is often an "all or nothing" process. An alternative is mediation, where a mediator attempts to craft an agreement addressing the needs and obligations of both parties. Mediation usually is less contentious and more efficient than litigation.

If our care and difficulties are ongoing, our claims adjuster may want us to settle our cases. Settling our case means our employer and/or our employer's insurer makes us a payment covering existing medical and work-loss expenses and absolving them of any potential future liability for our problem. Some settlements may keep medical benefits open or set aside an amount to allow us to seek medical care in the future. Settling the claim before the full extent and duration of our problems are completely understood is a gamble—and we will generally have far less information than our employer or our employer's insurer will have available about these kinds of gambles. Settlements may be in a lump sum or payable over time.

We also need to be aware that if companies try to close out our entire claim, including medical, we may be facing additional issues. In the United States, the Medicare and Medicaid programs are often "secondary payers"—meaning they may provide additional compensation after our primary insurers end our coverage. The U.S. government now has rules preventing shifting financial responsibility from a workers' compensation claim onto federal programs. These programs may require setting aside a portion of any settlement to cover the government's possible future exposure.

When we have a work-related problem we deserve appropriate care and compensation, including compensation for loss of wages and any permanent injury. Ideally this is what the "system" is supposed to do. We must be attentive to the process and be aware of the challenges we may encounter.

Vehicle Insurance Compensation

Vehicle insurance is primarily liability coverage for negligent acts or omissions using vehicles that cause death, bodily injury, and/or property damage. Other elements of vehicle insurance address comprehensive loss and/or collision damage for our vehicles.

In the United States vehicle insurance is divided by our state laws into states having policies for which all compensation is based on findings of drivers being "at fault" versus states having policies for which compensation is, at least initially, based upon "no fault" coverage. About three-fourths of U.S. states mandate strictly "at fault" vehicle insurance while the remaining states have various forms of "no fault" insurance programs. States having policies for which compensation is initially based upon "no fault" coverage make allowances for "at fault" determinations if injury claims exceed a specified dollar amount or meet other requirements. Some states may also have provisions for personal injury protection (PIP) where care is provided to injured parties, without consideration of fault, up to specified limits.

Vehicle accidents range from those that barely leave a paint scratch on a car to those involving deaths and serious injuries. Important issues with vehicle casualty claims include what actual injuries are associated with the vehicle accident, what diagnostic studies and care may be required, and what level and type of permanent impairment or disability, if any, the accident may have caused.

If we are involved in a vehicle accident where we or someone else is injured we want to first assure that any injuries are promptly treated with the appropriate medical care. In the most serious accidents emergency medical care is usually summoned to the scene. We or other seriously injured individuals will first be medically stabilized and then promptly transported to the nearest available trauma center. In accidents involving significant but less severe injuries we may go to emergency medical facilities for immediate care. If the accident has not resulted in injuries needing immediate emergency care we are generally best advised to seek follow-up medical attention from our primary care doctors.

Multiple factors determine the likelihood, type, and severity of bodily injury following a vehicle collision. The strength and elasticity of tissues (muscles, tendons, ligaments, bones, etc.) and their ability to resist external stresses will influence our treatment, possibility of disability, and any permanent impairment. When we are young and at our most flexible we are less likely to be injured or to be seriously injured than when we have become older and less flexible.

Arguably the most important factor in injury from a vehicle accident will be the intensity and duration of any acceleration to which we have been subjected. The greater the acceleration and the longer it lasts the greater our chance of injury. The greater the damage to our vehicles— often the most obvious sign of acceleration intensity and duration—the more likely we are to be injured. The consensus of accident research looking at our injuries is that (assuming we are healthy and restrained by our seat belt, we are sitting in a normal position, and we have a head restraint) a single exposure to a rear impact of 5 miles per hour or less is unlikely to injure us. Accidents at higher speeds or involving other portions of the vehicle are more likely to hurt us.

If we suspect we may have sustained a back or neck injury we want to be careful about who we choose to see for medical care. Injuries may range from mild (neck pain) to catastrophic (such as a spinal cord injury and/or paralysis).

With only a mild neck-pain injury, such as most injuries described as "whiplash," we will typically see significant improvement within days and all the treatment we may need is some informed reassurance, a mild pain reliever (such as acetaminophen—commonly sold as Tylenol®), and some range-of-motion exercises. In the United States "neck-pain injuries" typically receive far more treatment than can be justified by our best scientific studies. Much of this treatment does us little, if any, good but can be highly profitable for our healthcare providers.

If we have a sore or stiff back or neck following a vehicle accident, it is perfectly reasonable for us to see a doctor for an evaluation. This is especially true if the accident was more severe and/or we have problems other than spinal pain. However, we want to remember that most spine pain will resolve within days. If we are recommended or prescribed extensive medications or treatments such as manipulation, massage, or physical therapy, we really want to carefully consider whether these medications and/or treatments are for our physical benefit or for the healthcare provider's financial benefit.

Power of Support

Caroline Sylva was forty-two when she was on Maui in Hawai'i helping her parent's elderly neighbor clean his house. The neighbor's wife had recently died and he needed assistance with laundry and cleaning.

After Sylva had finished cleaning some windows she went inside to put her cleaning supplies away. She was just leaving the house, standing on the entrance steps, when her parent's neighbor came home from his doctor's appointment. While the neighbor was driving up to the house he apparently stepped on the gas pedal instead of the brake pedal and drove right into Sylva.

Sylva's left leg was severed below the knee as the car pushed her into the house. She was taken to the nearest Maui emergency room for immediate treatment and then flown to Honolulu (on O'ahu, Hawai'i) for additional treatment.

Sylva was initially upset about the accident. She wasn't angry at her neighbor—she recognized it was an accident. She was grateful she was still alive.

She first found dealing with the compensation system and the insurance company scary—especially while she was still trying to adjust to the fact she'd just lost her leg. Sylva worked for a personal-injury law firm and, fortunately, they were able to help educate her on her possible choices of action. She decided not to begin with a lawsuit—all she wanted was to be fairly compensated for her losses and future needs.

In her early interactions Sylva was frustrated with the insurance company when they reported they would cover only ten thousand dollars—the limit of her neighbor's personal injury protection policy. Sylva's treatment costs exceeded that amount within the first week of her amputation.

The insurance company then involved an experienced case manager to help determine Sylva's current costs and what her needs and associated costs would be in the future. The insurance company accepted the life-care plan developed by Sylva and the case manager. While it had taken determination from Sylva, advice and education from her law-firm coworkers, and help from the case manager, the insurance company later became more cooperative.

Sylva did not want an excessive settlement—she just wanted to be treated fairly.

Sylva found that her family, doctor, case manager, coworkers, and, most importantly, her attitude helped her to get past this tragedy. Reflecting on her experience, she found that having a supportive husband and family was important in her recovery. Her husband and family reassured her and helped her maintain a positive attitude. Sylva feels that her family upbringing helped her deal with her situation.

Her doctor assured her that she would be OK and would be able to walk again. Her case manager encouraged her to keep going, tackling her problems one step at a time. All of these factors—her supportive family, doctor, and case manager; the advice and education from her law-firm coworkers; and her own determination and positive attitude—provided Sylva with the opportunity for a positive outcome. She was not trapped by anger and is grateful she is still alive.

Personal Injury Compensation

Personal injury is a legal term for an injury to body, mind, or emotions. Beyond injuries at work or involving vehicles, we may be injured as a result of accidents elsewhere. We may slip and fall, be assaulted, or be injured by defective products. We may be harmed by medical or other forms of negligence.

Depending on the intent or negligence of the responsible party, we may be entitled to monetary compensation from a party through a judgment or settlement. Damages may include emotional distress, loss of consortium, and pain and suffering. Unless the party responsible for the injury willingly assumes responsibility, we will likely need a lawyer to help us navigate the legal system to address these issues.

Private Disability Insurance

Many employers will provide us with disability insurance and/or we may also buy such insurance on our own.

We can get policies insuring us for short-term (three-to-six months) and/or long-term compensation. Long-term compensation will pay us a percentage, usually 50–60 percent, of our regular income for as long as we are disabled—usually until we reach age sixty-five. Each policy will have specific language about our requirements to receive compensation. Some policies will provide compensation if we cannot perform our usual occupation while others will only provide compensation if we cannot perform any occupation. Many policies may also provide us compensation if we become partially disabled. These policies may make up a portion of the difference between what we once earned and what we may later earn.

If we face a disabling condition the disability insurer will have us file an application for compensation. Documentation from treating doctors will be required. Our doctors' documentation will be reviewed and we may be required to submit to an independent medical evaluation before possibly receiving any compensation.

Many more of us will need short-term disability compensation than will need long-term compensation. If we have a qualifying injury or illness, short-term disability insurance pays us a monthly percentage of our gross income up to our contracted maximum time, typically six-to-twelve months.

Jon Seymour, MD, a leading U.S. expert on disability guidelines, offers the following about short-term disabilities:

> We are far more likely to return to work if we can shorten our absence from work. Short-term-disability work absences may often be significantly reduced through the use of evidence-based and data-driven medicine.
>
> We may have more opportunity for rapid, decisive medical care when we are covered by short-term disability insurance than we do when we are covered by workers' compensation. The complex legal requirements and competing agendas of workers' compensation often slows our access to medical care.
>
> Given the seriousness of our not returning to work, and our crucial advantages in quickly addressing medical problems, we need to treat short-term disability absences exceeding the recommended "minimum duration" as medical emergencies. All of the stakeholders— doctors, employers, case managers, and us and our families—should be communicating with each other. We want to use disability duration and treatment guidelines to help all of the stakeholders focus on our return to work within our "optimum duration" period.
>
> Our treating doctors should be fully informed about our work duties. Our employers should be helping and encouraging our return to work by offering duties scaled to our increasing capacities. Our case managers should be coordinating this effort in a professional manner. We want to stay positive and stay focused on our rapid return to productivity.

At the end of our short-term disability compensation we might, depending on our condition and the language of our insurance policies, access long-term disability compensation.

Lester Kertay, PhD, one of the leading U.S. experts on long-term disabilities, offers the following:

> When injury or illness restricts our ability to work we need to remember private disability insurance is only intended as a safety net preventing catastrophic financial loss. The purpose for such insurance

is to provide us help while we must be away from our jobs—and to help support our getting back to our jobs as quickly as we can.

It will be a particularly difficult time for us to try and understand complicated contracts and deal with insurance requirements for medical records and employer information. We will find ourselves away from our jobs—and missing our paychecks—while we are focused on dealing with our injury or illness and trying to get better. But navigating our insurance system in a non-adversarial way is important—it offers us our best chance to get the help we need when we need it.

What help we may or may not get from our disability policies will be determined by the definitions and requirements contained in our contracts.

Sometimes we may be happily surprised to find our insurance offers us help going even beyond regular financial payments. It is important for us to identify and understand what additional help our insurance may offer us.

Often disability policies will offer employee assistance programs helping us with our, and our family's, emotional and personal stresses during these difficult times. We may also have rehabilitation benefits available to help us return to our jobs—either with our prior employer or with another employer. If we cannot continue to work in our earlier field, we may get retraining help to enable us to find new jobs in other fields.

Sometimes, even if we are hurt, because of the definitions and requirements of our contracts, help will not be available to us—even though it seems to us as though it should be. Being refused help we believe we deserve can be frustrating and can easily lead to adversarial relationships with our insurers. If we are initially refused help, we believe we deserve we can always ask for further, and higher level, reviews of our situations.

Just as with all of our other challenges in coping with and recovering from our injuries or illnesses, we need to stay as proactive and positive as possible. We need to approach our claims adjusters with cooperative attitudes. We are most likely to build collaborative relationships through cooperation. When we are able to address our issues cooperatively we may even find we can see beneficial changes in initial assessments and early conclusions.

Collaborative relationships will help us find security in our understanding of our insurance and make it easier for us to receive all the help we deserve. We want to feel certain our claims adjusters, and the companies they represent, share our goal of returning us to higher levels of functioning just as quickly as possible.

Americans with Disability Act

The Americans with Disabilities Act of 1990 (ADA) is a wide-ranging civil rights law prohibiting, in specified circumstances, discrimination based on disability. As defined by the ADA, disability is "...a physical or mental impairment that substantially limits a major life activity." "Covered entities," such as larger employers, are prohibited from discriminating against qualified individuals with disabilities. For those of us who are disabled the ADA mandates improved access to commercial facilities, employment, government services, public accommodations, and transportation.

Social Security

In the United States the U.S. Social Security Administration provides retirement and disability compensation as well as other forms of assistance. Social Security Disability Insurance is the leading safety-net program for America's disabled workers.

If we have an injury or illness interfering with our ability to work, and if we do not have private disability insurance, it may be appropriate for us to apply for Social Security Disability Insurance. Our applications may be made in person at Social Security offices, by phone, or online. We will need to complete an adult disability report and provide an authorization for our healthcare providers to disclose our medical information.

Our medical records will be obtained and our state Disability Determination Services will review our claims and make a decision. Their decision may take as little as one month or as long as several months. Initially most applications for disability compensation will be denied. On appeal many denials are reversed and compensation will be awarded.

Over the last three decades there has been a marked increase in our disability compensation claims. A larger workforce, a weakening economy, lowered eligibility standards, and an aging workforce all seem to be contributing factors. In 1990 there were three million recipients, in 2007 there were a little over seven million recipients, and by 2011 there were eight-and-a-half million recipients receiving Social Security Disability Insurance. Most enrollees in 2010 named either back pain or mental problems as their disabling injury, compared with only 26 percent making such claims in 1965. Both of these ailments are among the hardest to medically evaluate—which may potentially increase fraudulent claims.

Richard Burkhauser, professor of policy analysis and management at Cornell University, testified before Congress. He stated that Social Security Disability Insurance is often used as a long-term unemployment program for those of us who could be participating in the workforce if we had the appropriate workplace accommodations and rehabilitation.

A Social Security program called "Ticket to Work" offers those who are between eighteen and sixty-five and are receiving Social Security Disability Insurance or Supplemental Security Income greater opportunities for receiving employment services. Under this program the Social Security Administration issues "tickets" to those eligible so that we may, in turn, assign our "ticket" to an employment network of our choice to obtain employment services, vocational rehabilitation services, or other support services we may need to achieve our vocational goal. The employment network accepting our "ticket" provides and coordinates services matched to our needs to help us find and maintain employment.

Veterans and Wounded Warriors

The U.S. Department of Veterans Affairs (VA) uses its own schedule for rating disabilities. Determining compensation for those of us who are veterans is an exceptionally complex process.

According to the 2009 American Community Survey, in the United States an estimated 17.5 percent out of roughly 12,600,000 of us who are non-institutionalized civilian veterans aged twenty-one to sixty-four reported having a service-connected disability. Of those, an estimated 20.3 percent reported having a 70 percent or higher VA disability rating.

More military veterans returning from Middle East deployments will only increase the number of disabled veterans. Military-service members are entitled to receive expedited processing of disability claims from the Social Security Administration.

Paradoxically, many of us who are wounded warriors with the most severe losses, including losses of limbs, spinal-cord injuries, and post-traumatic stress disorder, do not perceive ourselves as disabled.

8

Healers

I started off thinking my doctors were responsible for my health.
Now I see only I can be responsible. My doctors work for me.
I am getting smarter in deciding who I will allow to be involved in my medical care—and what care I will allow.
Knowing I am in charge and responsible feels great— and I just keep on getting better.

What Do We Need?

Why do we see healthcare providers? We seek care for emergencies like broken bones or something scary like unexplained chest pains. We seek care when we are worried or our discomfort rises past our personal threshold.

How do we choose the healthcare provider best for us and our needs? How do we know if the care provided us is the right care? Often it can be tough.

We want our healthcare providers to help us maintain and, when needed, help us restore our health. We want them to focus on our ability to function, to diagnose us accurately, and, if we need it, to provide the treatment we require.

We want treatment consistent with the best and most current evidence-based medicine. We want treatment guided by our doctor's understanding of the "biopsychosocial" (relating to the interrelation of biological and social factors and our individual thoughts and behaviors—in contrast to strictly biomedical aspects of disease) perspective. We do not want treatments supported by someone's personal opinions or best guesses—and we especially do not want treatments based on what makes the most money for the healthcare provider, pharmaceutical companies, or others.

Our health is always our own responsibility. While we may seek help from healthcare providers *we* need to stay in control. Our healthcare providers must work with us. *Our* most important contribution is to *always* be active in maintaining our health.

Most of us do not spend much time thinking about health—until we start thinking something may be wrong. Then we start wondering how serious it might be. We consider our symptoms. If our symptoms are mild and do not last long, we usually try to take care of them on our own, often just by waiting for them to go away.

We consider if we are seeing things that are signs of serious problems—such as sudden and significant unexplained weight loss or blood in our urine. Some changes are so obvious we do not need any particular training to know they mean something is wrong—even when we might not have any idea what our problem might be.

If we want to know more about our symptoms we may stop by our bookstore or our library seeking references or look electronically for reliable resources on the Internet. A list of recommended Internet resources may be found in the back of *Living Abled and Healthy* and is available at www.livingabled.com.

We need to be careful about where we look for information. Books and Internet resources may offer us as many—or even more—opportunities for bad information as they do for good information. Often the best resources will be those provided by the government or by major medical schools or respected research hospitals. We want to be suspicious of any resource—print or electronic—trying to sell us medications or other treatments or funded by companies trying to sell us these things.

We may seek help from medically knowledgeable relatives or friends. If we can get suggestions from more than one knowledgeable relative or friend, we may be lucky enough to find the same suggestion offered more than once. If we get the same suggestion offered more than once, it will often be our best place to start.

When a medical problem persists or gets worse we need to see a healthcare provider. If we already have a primary care doctor, this would usually be our best first choice—unless the problems become so urgent we need to immediately go to an emergency room or even call an ambulance. We're better off when we can see healthcare providers *before* problems become emergencies.

The information in this chapter and later in "Diagnosing and Treating" will help us explore different healthcare providers, how problems are best diagnosed, and common treatments. We need to know as much as possible to stay as healthy as we can.

Who Comes First?

We would like to be able to always trust healthcare providers and have total confidence they always act in our best interests.

While mostly true, unfortunately this is not always true. Care in selecting the right provider is important. Some healthcare providers may generate more problems than help. Medical bias, lack of experience, lack of knowledge, or limited or dated skills can all cause problems. Problems may stem from healthcare systems prioritizing speed of patient contact over quality of care or, for some, simply greed.

We may more likely encounter less objective healthcare providers when we deal with work-related, vehicle, or personal injuries. Although many excellent providers focus on such injuries, questionable providers are also drawn to these kinds of injuries. Questionable providers may see such injuries as easy income opportunities as they may face fewer restraints treating insured injuries than those faced in general healthcare.

Because insured injuries often generate legal actions requiring lawyers, sometimes we may leave our usual primary care doctors. Many primary care doctors do not want to deal with the processing of such claims—which often including dealing with forms, depositions, letters, and testifying in court.

We may become involved with specialist doctors who appear to be aligned with the plaintiffs (the injured parties—us) or the defendants (employers and/or insurers). Some specialists may generally be more accepting of one side of a claim or litigation or the other.

These doctors are not necessarily biased based on who is paying them. Rather, their concepts and approaches may be more aligned with the interests of either plaintiffs or defendants.

Plaintiff's lawyers may prefer to work with doctors who more typically attribute problems to an injury, evaluate problems as more severe, recommend and provide extensive treatment, and provide higher impairment and disability ratings. Defendant's lawyers may prefer to work with doctors who are less likely to attribute problems to an injury, evaluate problems as less severe, recommend and provide minimal treatment, and provide lower impairment and disability ratings. Ideally we want to work with doctors who are skilled and unbiased.

We need to develop our own resources to distinguish good, evidence-based medicine from bad medicine.

Maximizing Benefits From Healthcare Providers

We need to take charge of our healthcare and make sure our healthcare providers offer us their best support. Maximizing the value of healthcare visits requires planning and action *before* we actually see our providers. Waiting until we are at the office will leave us rushed and maybe intimidated and we probably won't remember everything we thought was important.

Resources and forms making it easier for us to control our office visits are available at www.livingabled.com. Printing and then *using* these tools will help us take control and get the kind of advice and treatment we need.

"Doctor Visit" forms focus us on dates and times of our appointments, reporting changes in our health and/or conditions, and listing healthcare concerns. Offering our doctor a record of other healthcare providers we've seen, medications (including prescribed, over-the-counter, natural, and herbal and dietary supplements) we've taken, life situation and/or lifestyle changes, and our specific questions will make for more effective visits. On our first visit with a new doctor we want to bring with us all of our current medications in their original containers.

Before our first visit to a new doctor for an injury-related problem we should complete copies of the forms for the doctor and always keep extra copies for ourselves. Keeping extra copies for ourselves gives us a reference for what we reported and means we can always make additional copies for other providers or other purposes.

Helping our doctors only helps us. We want to be sure to arrive on time and to complete any other forms or questionnaires requested by the receptionist or nurse. Having our own forms already filled out will make completing a new doctor's forms much easier.

During our first visit with any new doctor we should talk with the doctor about what we expect.

We may offer a new doctor a copy of the "Patient-Doctor Agreement" and explain how this agreement describes the relationship we are seeking. We can ask our new doctor if they would review the agreement before our next visit and, if they agree, then sign it with us.

Using a "Patient-Doctor Agreement" may be new to some doctors—it will not be new to many primary healthcare doctors. Quality doctors should not find our requests threatening. If we meet a new doctor who seems threatened or appears irritated by our requests, we may want to consider seeing another doctor.

When visiting new doctors we should expect that our doctors will take a complete medical history. When we tell our stories we want to start by talking about our biggest concern—our "Chief Complaint." We then need to tell our stories from the beginning, explaining our history step by step, and how our bodies and lives have changed over time.

Even though we have told our stories before to other doctors we must expect to tell them again to each new doctor we see. If we forget to include *all* of the parts of our stories *each time,* doctors may miss important information or be misled or become concerned when our stories are compared to our other medical records. This is one more way our having completed copies of the forms with us will make our lives easier and help us tell our stories accurately and consistently.

We want to talk about our symptoms by telling how they have affected our daily lives. If the problem is on one side of our body—possibly one arm or one leg—we can compare the problem side to the side without problems. Even when we are asked "yes or no" questions we can always feel free to offer additional information.

If we become concerned our doctors are not listening carefully to what we are saying we need to express our concerns. We need to demand that our histories be listened to with attention. Especially if we are being rushed and when we view doctors as intimidating and more knowledgeable and more powerful than ourselves this can be difficult. But it is something we must absolutely force ourselves to do.

Most diagnoses will be developed from our histories—so it is extremely important we make sure they are given proper attention. This will be easier when we offer clear, consistent, and well-organized histories.

Doctors will need to perform physical examinations. We want to dress knowing we will have to remove some clothing, or change into examination gowns, so our doctors can give us thorough examinations. If we are being examined by doctors of the opposite gender, we are entitled to ask for someone of our gender to be present during our examination.

If the problem is on one side of our body, we should expect our doctors will examine our opposite side for comparison. If we experience sensations, pain or tightness, for example, during our examination we should report these sensations. If we are asked to do movements, such as bending a joint or our spine, we should demonstrate our full capabilities. However we want to also tell the doctor if we experience any symptoms while performing those movements. We need to tell them whatever concerns or worries us. We are entitled to ask if they have found any abnormalities during our examinations.

After histories have been taken and physical examinations are completed, the doctor will develop a "differential diagnosis" (a list of possible diagnoses) with a "working diagnosis" (our most probable diagnosis).

We should ask about the diagnoses and not finish the office visit without being told what the doctor determined as our "working diagnosis." We need this explained until we fully understand what is being described. We should be told the relative likelihood of all of the different possible diagnoses for our differential diagnosis and how our "definitive diagnosis" will be determined.

When doctors recommend specific diagnostic testing we need to ask why, what the risks and benefits may be, and how the results of this testing will affect treatment. If the answer we are given is that our doctors "always" get particular tests for all patients, we should be concerned. If, for example, we have back or neck pain without substantial trauma and without "red flag" symptoms of potentially dangerous conditions, we should not expect the doctor to order x-rays on our first visit. Diagnostic testing should have logical reasons specific to our individual situations.

We should expect to work together to determine our diagnosis. We can question our possible diagnoses without questioning the doctors' judgments by asking "how" and "why" questions. We can reasonably expect doctors to explain what they know about our diagnosis and how we may learn more. We should feel free to continue to repeat what our major concerns or worries may be. When we do not understand what we are being told we need to continue asking for clearer explanations until we do understand.

Once we have a working diagnosis we may begin discussing treatment options. We should question the benefits and risks of various options. We may choose to ask what they would do if they or their family members were the patient. Decision-making must always be shared.

When our doctors suggest treatments profiting their practices, such as treatments performed in their offices or at affiliated locations, dispensing of medications and/or devices, or surgery, we want to ask ourselves whether the opportunity for added income may be influencing their suggestions.

The best patient-doctor relationships occur when there are clear and honest communications. We should expect to be treated with dignity and respect—and we must equally treat our doctors with dignity and respect. Even if we may sometimes feel frustrated and not enjoy our doctors' behaviors we need to remain courteous. When doctors respect us and like us we will receive better care.

Although it may be difficult, during visits we should take notes, write down the answers to our questions, note the names of the care team, and record what *we* need to do next. This will help us manage our visits so that we may receive better healthcare.

Healthcare Professionals

Our healthcare team includes aids, dieticians, doctors, nurses, nurse practitioners, physician assistants, social workers, spiritual counselors, therapists (mental, occupational, and physical), and others. Depending on our specific needs and the people we meet, we will find some of these individuals more helpful in our recovery than others.

Primary Care Doctors—Our primary care doctor, if we have one (and, if we possibly can, we always should), will be someone who knows us, our medical history, our current and past medications and treatments, our personalities, and our values. Primary care doctors typically educate us regarding healthy lifestyle choices, provide preventive medical care, assess the urgency of problems, identify and treat common problems, and, when necessary, provide referrals to qualified specialists.

We choose a primary care doctor often by first asking medically knowledgeable relatives or friends for their recommendations. We may also seek recommendations from other healthcare professionals we already know and trust such as our dentists or pharmacists. We can look for information from our health plans, state medical associations, or advocacy groups.

In choosing a primary care doctor we want to consider their training and qualifications; specialty-board certifications; participation in healthcare plans; and availability by location, patient loads, and schedules. We may also evaluate the friendliness and helpfulness of their office staffs and what medical colleagues and other patients have to say about them. We want a primary care doctor who involves us as a full partner in our medical care.

There is a growing abundance of websites inviting anonymous posted ratings of doctors and other service providers from accountants to zoologists. Sometimes, if we see consistent comments about a healthcare provider, we may wish to consider the comments offered— but isolated comments are meaningless and often such sites may be posting biased information.

Specialists—For certain problems primary care doctors will recognize the limits of their expertise and they may refer us to specialists. While we want to strongly consider specialists suggested by our primary care doctors, we still want to do our own research on specialists just as we have on our primary care doctors. A checklist to help us identify our best choices of doctors is available at www.livingabled.com.

If our problems are work-related, occupational medicine doctors may be an appropriate choice. These specialists are experienced in the evaluation and treatment of work-related conditions. They will likely be able to assist us in staying at or returning to our jobs.

For many pain problems, particularly those involving muscle or nerve injuries, physical medicine and/or rehabilitation doctors may be appropriate choices.

If our problem is clearly related to our bones, the first choice would likely be an orthopedic surgeon.

If our problem involves our brain or nervous system, appropriate care would probably be provided by a neurologist or a neurosurgeon.

Nurses, Nurse Practitioners, and Physician Assistants—Doctors work with numerous other professionals to manage our acute and chronic medical conditions.

Nurses are often able to spend more time with us, relating to us, understanding our situations, and explaining our treatments. They are often our best access point into the healthcare system. Nurse practitioners are advanced-practice registered nurses with additional knowledge, skills, and training. Physician assistants are licensed to practice medicine as part of a healthcare team including doctors. In many practices, physician assistants will serve as our primary contact.

Physical and Occupational Therapists—Physical therapy focuses on promoting and restoring functional abilities so we may participate as fully as possible in our lives. Physical therapists are involved with preventing, evaluating, and managing our impairments, functional limitations, and disabilities relating to our health, function, and movement. Occupational therapy has a slightly different focus. Occupational therapy focuses on modifying our physical environment as well as training us to use assistive equipment to increase our independence. Both therapies are often combined to provide our treatment.

Physical and occupational therapists range from those with doctorates to physical or occupational therapy assistants and aides. Their approaches and techniques may vary widely.

Active "functional restoration" has been shown to be most effective for our muscle, tendon, and/or bone problems. Passive modalities such as electro-stimulation, heat packs, and ultrasound treatments should play a more limited role.

Treatment programs must start with careful physical evaluations and then develop plans dictated by our specific functional goals. We are likely to often need two or three therapy sessions a week and our between-visit exercises and other activities. Therapists should be educating us and making us responsible for our recovery.

We should be skeptical concerning the quality of care if

- the therapist does not communicate effectively or provide the attention we deserve;
- the treatment plan and specific measurable functional goals have not been fully explained and are not measured at regular intervals;
- the therapist is not empowering us to do more on our own;
- electro-stimulation, heat packs, or ultrasound treatments are used for longer than two weeks;
- the facility is owned by a doctor (especially if it is owned by our prescribing or referring doctor);
- we are not making steady progress.

Jaco Van Delden, a graduate of the Amsterdam Academy of Physical Therapy, Netherlands, and an experienced and well-regarded physical therapist, offers the following:

> Physical therapy may help us become confident and often upbeat when we have been unsettled and vulnerable. It will help us recognize that we are not alone in our recovery process. During physical therapy we may, consciously or unconsciously, communicate how we may be better treated in the future.
>
> We should expect physical therapists to ask about our difficulties and the challenges we face in living our daily lives. We should expect them to relate to how these affect our sense of well-being.
>
> We should expect physical therapists to consult with us concerning

our care plan and home exercise program. We should expect them to be attentive to our injuries and to use manual skills to help us resolve physical limitations. We should also expect them to help us to improve our current limitations in joints, muscles, ligaments, and nerves. We should expect physical therapists to help us to recover our independence sooner rather than later.

Mental Health Providers—In their haste to diagnose a physical cause for our suffering, some providers may overlook emotional or psychological issues. Our emotional or psychological issues may sometimes contribute to or be exhibited as physical symptoms. Anxiety, depression, or other psychological challenges may prolong and complicate our recovery from many physical conditions and place us at greater risk of developing disability. Emotional or psychological issues may sometimes lead to disability even when we have little or no physical injury, as in some cases when we experience depression or post-traumatic stress.

We may encounter social stigma associated with our experience of mental health challenges. Such social stigma is based on invalid stereotypes held by others and, in some instances, even by ourselves. These stereotypes are based on fears, popular misconceptions, and our lack of valid information.

Social stigma associated with an experience of mental health challenges can lead to belittling and trivializing behavior towards us and our problems. We must not allow social stigma to limit our willingness to seek support for treatable conditions.

Why should treating our mental health challenges be seen as different from treating our physical injuries or illnesses? All are sometimes aspects of who we are.

Steven and Norma Leclair, both PhDs and mental health professionals, offer the following guidance on when we should seek mental health services, how to select our appropriate providers, and how to determine if our care is what we need.

When should we consider mental health treatment? It is always important—if we believe we are facing mental health challenges—to begin addressing our concerns by first having a thorough physical examination to see if we have a physical disorder which may explain or contribute to our symptoms. Mental health treatment should be considered when we experience personal challenges involving anxiety; depression; the use of alcohol or other drugs or substances or activities to lessen our suffering; anger and irritability; long-term unresolved grief; or other similar sustained symptoms.

Treatment is particularly important when these challenges are serious, worsen over time, were once "manageable" but are now less so, or are affecting our ability to work, be successful in school, take care of ourselves or our families, or to enjoy any regular aspects of our lives. When the experience of anxiety, depression, or other mental health symptoms seriously affects our ability to function in our daily lives, we need to address it.

What about medication—when might that be helpful? If we are experiencing distressing or significant mental health symptoms, we may want to consider the use of psychotropic medications. Many primary care providers (including primary care nurse practitioners and physician assistants) are fully competent to recognize and treat our low-to-moderate mental health issues and are willing to prescribe and monitor the effects of psychotropic medications.

When our mental health problems become more serious or complex, a referral to a specialist in prescribing psychotropic medications—a psychiatrist, psychiatric nurse practitioner, or a physician assistant with a specialty in psychiatric care—should be considered. Depending on our location or community, the availability of prescribing specialists may be limited. It is always important that we feel comfortable with our prescriber and believe we are respected, listened to, and can be completely open and honest about our symptoms and other aspects of our experience.

How do I identify a therapist who fits my needs? Our choice of which therapist may be best to help *us* address *our* problems is critical.

Psychotherapy is an active, collaborative process where we seek support and guidance to alleviate our personal problems and help us grow as individuals. We must be ready to commit our time and energy to explore our thoughts, behaviors, and feelings. Our commitment will include regular attendance, honest disclosures, and follow-through with between-session homework. We will need to push ourselves to explore and share issues that may be hard for us to discuss.

Therapy should be considered as either our primary treatment or along with possible medication. Therapy can be particularly important when our mental health symptoms combine with a physical injury or illness and add more difficulties to our ability to function.

Similar to seeking any other specialist, we can start a search for a therapist by asking for suggestions from our primary care doctor or knowledgeable relatives or friends. We want to keep in mind that the personal experiences our relatives or friends may have had in counseling will reflect their perspectives so their suggestions may not necessarily fit our needs. Other people we can speak with include our clergy or local psychologists, clinical counselors, or clinical social workers.

Psychologists, clinical counselors, psychiatric nurses, clinical social workers, marriage and family therapists, pastoral counselors, and some psychiatrists provide counseling and psychotherapy services. Depending on our state or province, the above professionals should be licensed to diagnose and treat mental health problems. They also should have graduate degrees and have undergone supervised experience as a part of their training.

Our first questions should address their educational backgrounds, training, and licenses. Our second question should address what specialized training and/or experiences they may have had that would be helpful in addressing *our* problems.

The training and credentialing of therapists are typically not as important as we might want to believe. A doctoral-level therapist is not necessarily better than one with a master's degree. Our professional's therapy orientation and techniques also are not the strongest factors in success. Research consistently suggests that our engaging, open, positive, and trusting relationship with our therapist is the key to our counseling success.

Cognitive (knowledge based) behavioral therapy is an approach that may be helpful in dealing with our chronic pain. This approach addresses dysfunctional emotions and inappropriate behaviors and helps us improve the ways we think about our problems. These changes may be accomplished through a series of goal-oriented therapy sessions. Cognitive behavioral therapy is problem focused and action oriented. Goals are identified and our successful achievement of these goals is continually monitored and assessed.

Hospice-Care Providers—Hospice care may be provided at hospitals, skilled-nursing facilities, dedicated hospice centers, or even in our own homes. Hospice care is end-of-life care—usually defined as being for those of us who are not expected to live more than another six months and often for those of us whose lives are likely within weeks or even days of reaching completion.

Hospice staff are specialists in providing for our medical, psychological, and sometimes spiritual care, as well as support for our immediate family or close friends, at this critical final stage of our lives. As described by the National Cancer Institute, hospice caregivers "try to control pain and other symptoms so a person can remain as alert and comfortable as possible." "The goal of the care is to help people who are dying have peace, comfort, and dignity."

Complementary and Alternative Medical Providers—Many of us swear by the results of complementary and alternative medicine. Advocates of complementary and alternative medical therapies have often been previously disappointed by the failings of what we now consider traditional "Western" medicine.

Examples of complementary and alternative medical therapies include acupuncture and other aspects of traditional Chinese medicine; aural, electromagnetic-field, and other energy therapies; body manipulation; herbal medicine; homeopathy; and naturopathy. The important question is, as always, what really works?

Even beyond our concern with "what works," we need a concern with "what may be doing us harm?" While going through the existing governmental approval process is not a total guarantee of drug safety, the absence of such studies offers us even less information on the effectiveness, possible side effects, and possible interactions with other drugs—pharmaceutical or "natural"—of alternative remedies.

What do we recognize as the benefits of complementary and alternative medicine? One of the most cited benefits is the experience of providers' caring and concern—often contrasted with the lack of personal attention we now frequently experience in the delivery of Western medicine. We do receive therapeutic benefits from having our fears and worries about our problems listened to. Procedure-oriented Western doctors given ten-minute patient-visit schedules have little opportunity—and often little incentive—to listen to us.

However, scientific evidence indicates that most of the effect of complementary and alternative medical therapies is placebo based—its direct effect is in our minds rather than in our bodies. Biostatistician R. Baker Bausell is the past research director of the National Institutes of Health-funded Complementary and Alternative Medicine Specialized Research Center. His studies demonstrated that, at least temporarily, the placebo effect of complementary and alternative medicine is capable of reducing pain. Bausell identified a plausible biochemical mechanism of action for the pain reduction from complementary and alternative medical therapies based on our body's internal opioid system. This is when the body is stimulated to produce pain-reducing chemicals similar to the narcotic opioid drugs often prescribed us for pain relief.

Beyond the effects of placebo medication, Bausell found no credible evidence suggesting any complementary or alternative medical therapy benefited existing medical conditions or reduced any medical symptoms. Nor does complementary or alternative medical therapy have a scientifically plausible biomechanical mechanism of action beyond that of a placebo.

Critics of complementary and alternative medicine have defined complementary and alternative medicine as a "set of practices that cannot be tested, refuse to be tested, or consistently fail tests." Most complementary and alternative therapies have so far lacked consistent scientific evidence to accurately assess their medical effectiveness— so their effectiveness has neither been proven nor disproven. When new therapeutic approaches are demonstrated to work they become incorporated—although sometimes slowly and frequently with significant resistance—into standard medical practices and are no longer considered "alternative."

Those of us who have unconventional somatic conditions—often undiagnosed even after our seeing multiple specialists of Western medicine—may, consciously or unconsciously, be seeking any diagnosis we can believe is scientifically valid. We may reject any suggestions that our "condition" is not identifiable by currently available objective scientific findings.

While some complementary and alternative medical treatments may have harmful side effects, often the greatest danger in our using these treatments is that such treatments may result in our possibly delaying available and effective traditional Western treatments. Before seeking complementary or alternative medical answers we really want to explore the most current evidence-based medicine to see if these treatments may help us.

Chiropractors—Back and neck pain is our most common complaint. Because of this, most of us are likely to someday encounter chiropractors. Many chiropractors really seem to—and do—care about us. We, however, need to look closely at what they do and ask, "Does this actually help us?"

When we experience low-back pain lasting a couple of days or longer we may go to a chiropractor for a spinal manipulation. Often within hours we may feel better. At least we think we are better—although frequently a bit sore.

Some scientific studies have suggested that spinal manipulation is one answer (others include exercise, massage, and physical therapy) providing us some relief from low-back pain. National practice guidelines suggest we might want to try this answer up to—but typically not more than—six times for a particular complaint.

Earlier we identified the Cochrane Collaboration as establishing the gold standard for evidence-based medical practices. Working from the limited number of scientifically recognized studies, the Cochrane Database Systematic Review found spinal manipulative therapy no

1

more effective for sudden and severe low-back pain than doing nothing. Other peer-reviewed studies (those formally evaluated by others with recognized competence in the specific area of study) have failed to convincingly demonstrate that these treatments benefit any ailment. At best, the results from spinal manipulative therapy are comparable to other forms of physical therapy. There is a lack of solid evidence that spinal manipulative therapy works for neck pain.

Spinal manipulative therapy is also practiced by other doctors and physical therapists. Practitioners apply force to a part of our spine where movement is reduced. Manipulation may produce popping noises from a reduction of the pressure inside our joints. The goal is to relieve our pain and improve our ability to move and walk. It is relatively safe.

Some chiropractors may find that our bones may be out of place (subluxations) and must be put back into proper alignment (adjustments). No one has ever scientifically proven the existence of a chiropractic subluxation. Even among chiropractors there is no consistent definition of "chiropractic subluxation." No evidence shows we need multiple adjustments to "stabilize" or "correct" our subluxations.

Chiropractic doctor and Health Science (evidence-based healthcare) PhD Preston H. Long wrote about chiropractic in his 2002 book *The Naked Chiropractor: Insider's Guide to Combating Quackery and Winning the War Against Pain* and again in his 2013 work *Chiropractic Abuse: An Insider's Lament*. Long offers the following:

> Chiropractic is a complex fabrication of many treatment techniques, belief systems, and marketing schemes. If a neighbor, close friend, or relative were to ask me, "How do I pick a chiropractor?" I would offer the following advice.
>
> If their problem was neck pain I could not in good conscience or with good science recommend a chiropractor under any circumstances. The inherent admitted risk of stroke following cervical manipulation greatly outweighs any personal belief in benefit.
>
> There is a lack of peer-reviewed clinical studies in support of spinal manipulation being helpful for any condition including

the cervical spine. Until these studies are performed and support spinal manipulation as a safe and beneficial treatment modality recommending its use is impossible.

If the problem resided in their mid- or low-back then a visit or two to the chiropractor might be a reasonable approach. Middle and lower backs are large structures well protected by ribs, deep spinal muscles, scapulas, and clavicles, just to name a few. If chiropractic treatment works it will work in one or two visits, maybe three—ten or more are never needed.

I would not encourage chiropractic if a neurological sign or symptom was being experienced, such as pain shooting down the back of the leg. The medical community is far better trained and equipped to diagnose neurological disorders than an average chiropractor.

I would also inform them that they should be given an informed consent form detailing the recommended care, the risks associated with chiropractic, costs, alternatives, and the natural resolution of their problem.

If they were diagnosed with subluxations I would have them leave the office and not return. Subluxations are mythical entities that never require treatment. I would advise them against monthly maintenance care, as that has not been shown to be beneficial except to the chiropractor's bottom line.

Simply stated, if a neighbor, close friend, or relative came to me with back pain I would never think or say: wow you need to see a chiropractor right away. I cannot think of a single scenario where chiropractic would be my first recommendation.

A better question then might be: why would someone ever see a chiropractor?

We need to be particularly concerned if chiropractors wish to perform spinal manipulation under anesthesia. Refusal by a chiropractor to provide us with records or providing records that are difficult to understand would also be causes for concern.

Some chiropractors work closely with plaintiff's lawyers. Some lawyers who represent us when we have been hurt find it helpful for chiropractic providers and other doctors to demonstrate how injured we are. If we have received thousands of dollars of chiropractic care, then surely we must have been seriously injured. Both chiropractic providers and lawyers make money—but we may end up believing we are more injured than we actually are.

What does this mean for us? If we have sudden and severe low-back pain, we could give it a try. If we choose chiropractic care, we should expect to see a lessening in our pain and an improvement in our function in—at the longest—six visits. More treatment is unlikely to provide any additional benefit.

Healthcare Locations—We should try to be informed enough about our bodies and our medical issues to recognize the differences among our problems which may be handled by scheduled office visits, by urgent care centers, or those requiring emergency rooms or ambulance transport. Usually urgent care centers will allow more time to treat us and will cost us less than emergency rooms or ambulance transport.

If our problem is not an emergency and is work related, an occupational health clinic may be an excellent option. Occupational health clinics understand workers' compensation issues and most working environments. We should, however, be cautious about facilities advertising their focus as workers' compensation and vehicle-accident injuries.

9

Lawyers

I started out so ignorant about laws and lawyers. The
lawyers put out such reassuring advertisements.
Now I'm beginning to figure out when I need a lawyer
and when I don't.
When I decide I actually need a lawyer, I make sure
they know they work for me—and that I'll decide what
actions we'll take.

Advocates or Victimizers—or Both?

If we are significantly injured while working, involved in an accident
(particularly a vehicle accident), or become disabled, many of us will
enter a world of "wonder and worry." We will wonder and worry about
what has happened to us, what is going to happen to us, and what we
should do. We'll wonder whom we should trust.

The processes of claims and dispute resolution and litigation will
be confusing to most of us. Contemporary U.S. society has made all
Americans much too familiar with the idea of litigation—lawsuits.
But for the vast majority of us who are not professionally involved,
the actual process of litigation will be daunting and intimidating. As
untrained individuals, knowing we will be facing trained lawyers and
other trained professionals, most of us will see no option but to find
lawyers of our own.

Lawyers who represent us are known as applicant's, claimant's, and/
or, more generally, simply as plaintiff's lawyers. Lawyers who defend
employers and insurers are known as defense lawyers.

Plaintiff's lawyers may serve as effective advocates in helping us to secure care and compensation, particularly if we have faced barriers to access. Lawyers are legally and ethically obligated to represent their client's best interests—not their own. Sometimes there may be a real conflict between our best legal interests and our best medical interests. Our best legal interests may reflect our (and our lawyer's) financial compensation while our best medical interests may more generally reflect our long-term well-being.

Most lawyers are reasonable individuals interested in doing their jobs as they were trained. Legal training focuses our lawyers on "winning" as many cases as possible. In non-criminal cases (including injury and disability cases) the extent of "winning" is usually measured in the dollar value of the judgments or settlements secured. Legal training does not focus our lawyers on the quality of the lives led by their clients—us—after our cases are settled.

When we are injured, sometime after the questions concerning our immediate medical care have been resolved, we, and those who care about us, will often wonder "How much is this injury worth?" in dollars. We are also likely to be concerned about our possible need for longer-term medical care, how long we will have to be away from our jobs (and paychecks), and if we will be able to return to our jobs or another job (and paychecks). All of these concerns together may well drive us to consider our need for a lawyer.

In the United States we will not have to look hard to find a lawyer. We are drowning in ads by lawyers encouraging us to seek their help. Most lawyers specializing in injury and/or disability litigation will advertise "no fee unless recovery." In injury and/or disability litigation lawyers are most commonly paid on a contingency-fee basis where their income will be a portion (*before* "costs" are deducted—and costs may become a substantial percentage of a judgment or settlement) of whatever judgment or settlement is achieved. A few U.S. states provide injured workers public lawyers to represent their interests.

Contingency-fee arrangements are important. Contingency fees allow those of us with limited resources to file a claim or lawsuit against individuals, employers, or insurers with financial and legal resources vastly greater than our own when we believe we have been injured and we believe those other parties are responsible.

Usually our lawyer's contingency fee will be between 25 and 40 percent (*before* "costs") of whatever judgment or settlement is achieved. In reality, our lawyer's combination of costs and fees could potentially result in the majority of the settlement. Typically there is a "no win, no pay" arrangement—but, in most cases, we will still be responsible for costs such as court fees, filing fees, and paying for expert testimony.

Some plaintiff's lawyers may become more interested in their own financial gain than in their clients'—our—best long-term interests. This can include a technique of "churn 'em and burn 'em." This is where lawyers take as many cases as they can and try to settle these cases as quickly as possible for as much as they can get quickly—without extensive preparations and/or trials—so they maximize their hourly return. This may leave their clients—us—with only a fraction of the possible true value of judgment or settlement. Fast resolution may not be the best resolution for us.

Some lawyers will "cherry pick" only the strongest claims most likely to succeed with large expected judgments or settlements. This can make it difficult for us to get legal representation if our case has only a small dollar value—such as cases that include only limited medical bills. If our case includes both extensive medical bills and our inability to return to work, then the expected judgment or settlement will be much higher.

However, if our lawyer "wins" a case based on our inability to return to work then the judgment or settlement will be that we have become "disabled." Becoming labeled as disabled may significantly affect how we will be perceived by others and will almost certainly, in the long run, affect how we perceive ourselves. These changed perceptions are not likely to benefit us.

There is evidence that litigation makes it more likely we will take longer to heal and be more likely to become disabled. When cases have high medical costs, more permanent impairment, and result in permanent disability they will likely generate larger judgments or settlements.

All forms of claims and dispute resolution and litigation tend to drag on over many months and, most usually, multiple years. Medical treatments will almost always end up continuing throughout the process of our claims, dispute resolution, or litigation.

Some lawyers may encourage us to see doctors they know will frequently prescribe extensive drug and other treatments, sometimes including surgery. Sometimes lawyers may just be doing their best to get us to good doctors. We need to recognize, however, it is possible that lawyers are suggesting doctors who favor extensive medications and other treatments because larger medical expenses will likely result in larger fees for the lawyers. The more we are treated the more the expected judgment or settlement value of our case increases. The greater the value, the more money they make.

As injured patients we naturally want to get well as quickly as we can so we may resume our activities and return to our jobs. We are also entitled to seek the compensation we deserve.

Some lawyers will advise their clients to honor their doctor's advice and not resume activities or return to jobs until their cases are resolved—since resuming activities or working may reduce the expected judgment or settlement. At the same time as these recommendations are recognized as common legal practice, most lawyers are resistant to believing their recommendations may actually be causing harm to or generating disability in their clients.

Litigation is always being delayed. Lawyers may not have enough time to manage all their cases or the hearing venues may be overwhelmed. Delays can occur because of difficulties in getting appointments with doctors or obtaining information from doctors. Scheduling difficulties with hearings and courts will result in delays. The longer our case takes to be resolved the more likely we are to be harmed.

All of these litigation delays cause us significant stress—in addition to our concerns about healing. It only gets much worse if we are under financial pressures—which we usually will be when we are not at our jobs, not getting paychecks, and when those who care for us may also be losing time from their jobs to help us with our care and treatments.

The longer we are unable to resume our activities or return to work the longer we are learning to become disabled. When the opposing lawyers representing our employers or insurers question the legitimacy or severity of our injuries we may find ourselves forced to prove, over and over again, we are disabled. This becomes our "learned behavior"—

and we have earlier looked at just how critical our learned behaviors are to our physical realities.

When we involve lawyers in medical issues we surrender much of our personal control. Our lawyers, opposing lawyers, and hearing officers and/or judges now largely control our lives. To build their strongest legal cases our lawyers will develop and describe our worst possible physical cases. We may easily end up believing our worst possible physical cases will become our realities. This is, after all, exactly what our lawyers are trying to convince the opposing lawyers and hearing officers and/or judges will happen. The problem is that we may also believe these stories and therefore experience these outcomes.

Once our case is legally resolved, our lawyers expect to end their association with us and our medical problems. They are legal-services providers—not healthcare providers. They have no continuing legal or moral obligation to us past our legal judgment or settlement.

Choosing a lawyer is fully as difficult as choosing a good healthcare provider. Our first step, always, is determining whether we need a lawyer. We can follow the same paths we used to identify quality healthcare providers. If we already have a lawyer with whom we have worked and who we trust who practices in some other area of law, they may be able to suggest possible candidates. We can use Internet sites such as www.lawyers.com or www.findlaw.com for limited guidance. Our state and local bar associations usually offer referral services—but these provide little, if any, qualitative information.

Working with whatever resources we can identify, we need to narrow our list to two or three possible lawyers we may ask for initial consultations. For U.S. lawyers practicing in injury, disability, or workers' compensation law an initial consultation should typically be free. The lawyers we meet will assess our case and we will assess the lawyers. We want to ask if the lawyer specializes in our type of case, whether they have represented many others with similar situations, and whether they can represent us at all levels of the dispute-resolution process.

Before engaging a lawyer we should

- Do Internet research on our potential lawyers, determining if they have a website, a blog, are published, and the type of cases they focus on.

- Obtain information regarding their experience with our type of case. (Today this can most often be obtained by viewing the lawyer's website.)
- Ask them how many cases they have tried and what is their success rate?
- Assess whether the lawyer is a good listener, understands our case, and has a plan.
- Identify the lawyer's philosophy about our medical care and about our staying at or returning to our jobs.
- Try to develop a sense of what it would be like to work with the lawyer's office staff.
- Try to discern whether we can trust the lawyer.
- Obtain references and contact them.
- Review and understand the lawyer's financial arrangements, including such potential costs as accessing medical records, court reporters, or medical experts.

Knowing Who's the Boss

Robert Aurbach, an internationally known workers' compensation lawyer, offers the following:

> The most important thing we need to remember when we are dealing with a lawyer representing us is that our lawyer is our employee. Our case will be only one of many our lawyer is pursuing at one time so we cannot demand their full-time attention—but we are in control. A good lawyer will use their professional judgment and experience to advise and assist us but will follow our instructions, answer our questions, and respond to our communications in a reasonable time.
>
> It is incredibly easy for us to feel out of control when we are in a dispute about some part of our case. The language and rules controlling our case will be unfamiliar to us and we may be asked to do things we do not understand. The experience of injury comes with anxiety, physical discomfort, and, often, fear about our future. We are likely to be off work, away from many of the people we know, and we may be under financial pressure. It's easy at this point for us to simply fall into a pattern of doing whatever our lawyers, claims adjusters, or doctors tell us to do.

But it is dangerous for us to allow ourselves to lose our sense of control over the process.

Scientists tell us that when we are presented with multiple problems at the same time our brains process our incoming information by linking together whatever we are experiencing. Just as we might come to associate a song or a picture with other memories, our minds associate those things we experience at the same time. With repeated exposure (including our mental repetition, which happens when we repeatedly think about something), the connections in our brain become more automatic.

This is how we learn our habits, including our thinking habits.

When we are constantly presented with messages from the media and those around us about how we are victims, how helpless we are against larger interests, how little hope we have of regaining our former lives, and how getting money is our best way to make it all better, we have a serious problem. These inaccurate and negative thoughts become associated with our feelings of anger, anxiety, isolation, pain, lack of purpose, and, most importantly, being out of control—so when we feel any one of these things all of them come to mind together. This is how—and why—we learn to think of ourselves as disabled.

Some will say our injury is what disables us. This is true only in a small number of extremely severe cases. Our injury is what we have. Becoming disabled is one way—but not our only possible way—we may begin to think of ourselves in light of the injury.

The injury is not who we are unless we let others guide us into thinking this way. We all know of people (military wounded or stroke victims, for instance) who overcome significant physical challenges and resume happy and productive lives.

Lawyers often create conditions where they add to our messages of disability or create circumstances where our message of disability becomes our habit of thought. They seldom do this on purpose. They rarely even understand they are having a negative effect on how we will live our lives.

The first way our lawyers inadvertently harm us is by getting us to think we will be better off if we get a large judgment or settlement for our injuries. If our judgment or settlement comes at the expense of our losing our ability to make a living in the future, losing our access to our friends, or losing our self-respect and the respect of our family and friends, then the amount of any judgment or settlement we will get (especially from a limited statutory program like workers' compensation) will never be enough.

Yet that judgment or settlement usually becomes our lawyers' sole focus. The idea is fostered that maximizing the judgment or settlement on our case is the most important thing we need to consider. But medical research is clear that the longer we stay away from our jobs the less chance we have of ever returning to our jobs. And every workers' compensation system is designed to compensate us for less than we would make in our lives by returning to our jobs.

So our judgment or settlement, no matter how large, will never make us whole. Regaining our lives will make us whole. Workers' compensation is only designed to give us enough money to heal and get back to our lives as quickly as possible.

There are a number of other ways our lawyers inadvertently make their clients—us—helpless and contribute to our bad outcomes. Litigation is a long process. Most times we will probably never get "our day in court" to tell our stories and achieve any personal feeling of justice. Litigation is so expensive and time consuming that most cases will be settled before ever coming to a hearing or trial.

But we can still expect to invest months or years of our attention, our emotional energy, and our lives before we reach resolution while the system grinds through many other cases at the same time as ours. During this delay we may face anxiety, depression, and financial pressures. We will have far too much time getting used to others telling us what to do and far too much time for us to become comfortable with introducing ourselves to others as disabled. These habits will become hard for us to break.

If we've ever taken extended time off from work and found it hard to go back after our illness, layoff, pregnancy, or vacation was over, then we have experienced this problem before—but, by comparison, only in a minor way.

We will have far too much time, while our case is pending, for countless repetitions of all of the negative messages from the media and others. We will have far too much time to experience the different ways injured people are treated and repeatedly experience our own anxieties and fears. Over this far too much time, all of these various negative experiences will begin to seem normal to us.

Sometimes the words our lawyers (or our claims adjusters or the defense lawyers) use will begin to play over and over in our minds. "We will never be able to do our job again" is a strong message, as is questioning whether our injury occurred or whether we are really as hurt by it as we claim. The questioning of our integrity as a claimant is particularly difficult because it makes us "prove" we are disabled over and over again. And we all know that practice makes perfect.

While all this is going on our lawyers continue to treat us in ways which may not be beneficial to us. They may treat us as if we are disabled and unable to look after ourselves or make our own decisions. People will almost always begin to act the way we are treated—and our being treated as children unable to take care of ourselves will usually result in our childish behavior.

Our lawyer may try to protect us from our fears and the consequences of our actions in just the same way someone might "enable" the behavior of an alcoholic. Common experience tells us that when we are protected in this way we will seldom get better.

At the end of this process most often our lawyer will make a deal, usually with another lawyer with whom they have often dealt before and with whom they expect to deal again many more times. Our lawyer may be more interested in maintaining a good continuing working relationship with the opposing lawyer than in honoring our instructions as a one-time or occasional client. Any interest of our lawyer in our welfare generally stops when a deal is concluded.

After the deal is made our lawyer will no longer be there to advise or direct us. We must maintain our ability to take care of our own needs.

This is why it is so important to maintain our personal sense of control—so that when the time comes we will be able to pick up the pieces and get on with the rest of our lives.

Staying in control is hard. We must ask questions and make sure we get answers we understand. Knowledge is power. We want to keep in mind a bigger picture of what outcome we want to have for the rest of our life—not just for this claim—because what habits of thought we learn during this experience may come to define who we will be for the rest of our lives.

We must not be afraid to demand the time we need to make decisions. Sometimes it will be helpful for us to speak with someone we trust who has our best interests at heart but who is not involved in our claim in any way. If we always "keep our feet on the ground" by staying in control, we are more likely to be able to "hit the ground running" when our claim is resolved.

Winning is Everything—Or Is It?

David DePaolo, an experienced workers' compensation lawyer, is now president of WorkCompCentral, a resource for information on workers' compensation issues. Here are his thoughts on involving, selecting, and managing lawyers:

> Not all of our injuries or disabilities will require the assistance of a lawyer. But when we are dealing with complex, unfamiliar systems such as our state's workers' compensation laws or other specialized compensation protections there may be many times when we may find ourselves confused, overwhelmed, or in need of some help.
>
> The most important thing we need to remember when considering involving a lawyer is that our lawyer, in general, will only be paid if some disability (or similar) judgment or settlement is obtained in our favor. Thus our lawyer's incentive is aligned with our own only when we consider our finances—but this also means our lawyer's objective will always be to maximize our disability so as to maximize our judgment or settlement. While it will never be a problem for *our lawyers,* maximizing our disability may leave *us* with serious consequences down the road when we want to return to our jobs, find a new job, or face some subsequent injury.
>
> *When to Involve a Lawyer*—There is a difference between seeking counsel and obtaining legal representation.
>
> Seeking counsel is all about getting knowledgeable, trustworthy answers when we are confused, we do not understand the law, or we face multiple options and need some help in making our best decision.

Lawyers who work on a contingency-fee basis will generally be happy to provide us an hour or so of free consultation. But we need to understand this is not generosity or kindness, this is investigation and marketing for the lawyer. Lawyers will be using this time to determine whether they believe our case is likely to generate a sufficient financial return on their time investment (and fronting of costs) for them to take our case.

We may go in to visit a lawyer seeking counsel and come out having unintentionally committed to legal representation without even having gotten our questions satisfactorily answered. As has been said before, "There ain't no such thing as a free lunch."

We should obtain legal representation when we face a dispute or an adverse relationship we can recognize is beyond our ability to resolve on our own. This representation is the familiar and traditional role of our lawyers. When we have been injured and our injury was caused by another and they deny liability we will probably need a lawyer. When we have been injured in our workplace and we are not receiving prompt and appropriate medical care or our reasonable compensation is being delayed we will probably need a lawyer.

But we must always stay aware that once we have involved a lawyer in our case our lawyer's motivation will always be to maximize the financial aspect of our case. Sometimes maximizing the financial aspect of our case will conflict with our best interest in returning to our activities and our jobs as quickly as possible or of our quickly getting medical treatment that will actually help us to fully heal.

Selecting the Right Lawyer—Not all lawyers are equal! The law has many, many specialties and sub-specialties. Sometimes even a general personal-injury lawyer may not be our best choice.

When we are hurt at work we need to identify lawyers whose practice focuses on our state's workers' compensation system. Most U.S. states' bar associations recognize certifications of legal specialties. Workers' compensation law is generally identified as specialty law because workers' compensation laws and procedures are different from regular civil law.

Finding the right lawyer for our claim does not have to be hard but it will require us to do some work. Most state bar associations maintain websites with public listings of lawyers certified in various specializations. We can start there. We should also seek references from our knowledgeable relatives or friends or trusted professional associates.

The problem we will be facing is that all legal cases are different. The results someone else experiences with a specific case handled by a particular lawyer will not necessarily define the results we will see on our case. Sometimes we may even be happy with how one lawyer handles one case but unhappy with how the same lawyer may handle another case.

We want to try to identify three-to-five potential lawyers. Then we should call their offices to inquire about obtaining an appointment— but *not* actually set any appointments! The purpose of our first calls is just to gauge the responsiveness of different law offices so we can compare them against each other.

Law is a personal service and we want our lawyers to be responsive to our needs. Generally this means how often and how well they communicate with us.

Communication largely depends upon our lawyers' staffs—so our first calls are just to give us an impression of how responsive a law office may be. Are our calls being picked up immediately or are we placed on hold for transfers? If we leave messages, how long is it before we get a return call? If a secretary tells us our requested lawyer cannot immediately return our call, will the secretary find someone else who can answer our questions?

After we have narrowed our choices to two or three lawyers it's time for us to set consultation appointments.

We need to really *listen* to the lawyer's initial consultation advice about our case. This initial advice is called *managing our expectations*.

If a lawyer advises us that, based on their experience, our case does not merit their involvement, we certainly would not want to work with that lawyer even if they might be convinced to take us on.

If a lawyer advises us that, based on their experience, our case is probably not worth more than a certain amount, this lawyer is sending us an important message—that if we are expecting to see a larger judgment or settlement then getting this lawyer for our case is probably going to result in our being disappointed.

If one lawyer reviews our case and suggests that either our case does not merit their involvement or that any judgment or settlement might be small, it does not mean we should not get other opinions. If multiple lawyers offer similar opinions, we should seriously consider if this is a case we want to pursue.

If we meet with a lawyer and the lawyer offers an opinion concerning the value of our case which seems reasonable to us and is one the lawyer finds reasonable to proceed on, then we have identified a lawyer we want to seriously consider.

This stage is critical because, if our case is considered financially attractive (and most will be), once we are in the lawyer's office we will be pressured to sign an agreement with that lawyer that day.

Unless our case requires some emergency action on the part of a lawyer—which would usually mean *we* have procrastinated in addressing some legal obligation—we absolutely *do not* want to sign any agreement immediately.

We want to wait a day or more and review our notes about the different lawyers we have met and choose the one with whom we feel most comfortable.

Managing Our Lawyers—Once we are signed up with a lawyer or law firm the likelihood is that we will be handed off to support staff for most of our case. In general this need not be a bad thing—as long as our support staff is competent and can deal with our case.

But if we are not satisfied with our treatment from our support staff, then we need to make an appointment directly with our lawyer to discuss our concerns and see that our treatment changes until we are satisfied. If we were careful in our initial screening in our selection process, we should not face this problem.

We can never rely on the opinions of others who have had injuries we may think are similar to our own. We cannot allow the thoughts of others to steer our thoughts on our lawyer's work. All cases are different, no injury is the same, and even similar cases within the same system may have different outcomes based simply on the individuals involved. This is especially so if rules or laws have changed or even change midway through our case—which happens.

We also should *never* allow ourselves to feel pressured by our lawyers. Hard-sell tactics from our lawyers should be rejected—with a change of lawyers if necessary. At the same time, we must *always* honor our own responsibility to be reasonable.

The bottom line is that it is always *our* case and *we*, ultimately, have, and need to maintain, control. Being injured can be an emotionally trying time—being in litigation will almost assuredly be an emotionally trying time. Together they just feed upon each other and become more emotionally difficult.

When we are faced with critical decisions sometimes our best option is to take a day or two to collect our thoughts and temper our emotions before reaching our conclusion.

What Do We Do?

Sometimes we will need lawyers to help us; sometimes we do not. We can approach this decision the same way we considered medical treatments or drugs. There are specific indications for choosing to involve lawyers. We need to pay careful attention and we always need to consider the risks versus the benefits.

We may need lawyers when we have no other way to navigate litigation. Other times, however, we may be able to identify enough other sources of information to get by on our own. These alternative guides may include materials provided by our state, our employer, or our insurer. For workers' compensation cases our state may provide handbooks, websites, or even advocacy services. We may choose to represent ourselves, a situation called "pro se" or "pro per." If we represent ourselves we are required to abide by the same rules as lawyers, therefore we need to familiarize ourselves with statutes and rules.

In dealing with lawyers, as in dealing with doctors, we need to stay in control. There may come a time and a place in our lives for lawyers—but we are always best off to keep both our medical treatments and our legal treatments as simple as possible.

10

Other Players

*So many different people were getting involved in my
case I couldn't figure out who was doing what.
By stepping back and demanding explanations—
and not going forward until I understood what was
happening—I've now been able to understand what
everyone does and whether they're working for me or
working for someone else.
I'm better about getting accurate information and
recognizing when I don't yet have it.
I'm getting better at figuring out what I need and who
can help me get it.
Now my actions are based on what is right for me.*

Claims Professionals—Our Link to Successful Resolutions

The person in the most pivotal role in addressing our claim is the claims
adjuster or claims representative. The claims adjuster is the front-line
staff reviewing our claim and the individual responsible for handling
our claim from beginning to end. The job of claims adjusters is to
understand the state laws associated with our claim and process the
claim according to the regulations. The adjuster is knowledgeable about
the claims process from the filing to claim closure and will explain the
process and provide us a "road map" so that we understand what to
expect.

Our claims adjuster will interview us and others, investigate the
claim, and review our records. Decisions made by the adjuster will
profoundly affect us and the way in which our claim is processed.

We must always remember that the adjuster may initially approve or deny our medical treatments, disability compensation, or settlements. Adjusters may work for our large self-insured employers, insurance companies, or third-party claims-administration companies processing claims on behalf of an insurance company or employer. They face challenging situations in every claim they process and thoroughly review each claim.

Claims adjusters can be a resource for us when we have questions about compensation for ourselves or others—sometimes when we may be frightened and in pain, confused, and frustrated. They deal with our doctors and other healthcare providers wanting approvals and payments for drugs and other treatments. Possibly the most challenging for them, frequently adjusters must deal with lawyers.

While many insurance companies prefer claims adjusters who have four-year college degrees, the backgrounds of claims adjusters vary. Some states may require a state certification.

We are best off when we relate to our claims adjuster in a cooperative, honest, and respectful manner. We want them to be our allies. We do need, however, to always remember that our claims adjustors are working for the party we are expecting to pay our bills and compensation. There will always be some level of conflicting interests. If we are arrogant or threatening, we can expect the same lack of cooperation generated in almost all of us by others' arrogance or threats.

As with members of any profession, our claims adjusters may range from cooperative and friendly to rushed and having a bad day. Day in and day out they deal with many negative people in difficult situations. When we approach our claims adjuster in a positive manner we will stand out—and our claims adjuster will be more likely to assist us.

Kimberly George, senior vice president, senior healthcare advisor, Sedgwick Claims Management Services, offers guidance on relating to our claims adjusters:

> We should do our best to establish a positive relationship with our claims adjuster. Claims adjusters represent insurance companies or employers but they are also concerned about our well-being and want to be a resource for us regarding any questions we may have. Skilled

claims adjusters recognize their role is to provide us with appropriate compensation, to facilitate our healing, and to promote our return to work.

We should recognize it is better for us to establish a relationship with our claims adjuster as an ally rather than as an opponent. As with any relationship, our relationship with our claims adjuster works best when we have good communication, honesty, and trust. Our being polite and respectful will be more successful in achieving a positive outcome than our being demanding and rude. When our claims adjuster requests information we want to provide this information as promptly and as completely as possible. If a request is unclear, we need to ask for additional information. If we become uncomfortable with our relationship with our claims adjuster, we need to ask to speak with his or her supervisor and discuss our concerns.

Case Managers—Helping Us Navigate

We may be assigned a case manager to work with us. Case managers are typically assigned and paid by the insurer or by the employer at the request of the adjuster. The case manager's goal is to collaborate with us in assessing our needs and our situation, coordinating and planning our care, and facilitating the prescribed treatment plan. We will work together to, we hope, achieve a positive outcome. Many case managers may have nursing, vocational rehabilitation, or social-work backgrounds and many may have different certifications depending on their backgrounds and focus.

When we don't understand what is happening with our claim or we have complex medical issues, we can ask our claims adjuster or our lawyer (if we have one) to be assigned a case manager. Effective case managers work cooperatively with us and encourage our active involvement. We don't want and should never allow a case manager to assume primary responsibility for our care—we must always maintain our personal control.

Case managers need excellent listening skills. They serve as our advocates, facilitate healthcare communications, identify resources, and facilitate our medical care. Good case managers work with us to help us determine what we believe is important and our most effective answers to reach our goals. Mutual trust is needed for this relationship to be successful. Case managers are most effective when they facilitate direct communications among our employers, our healthcare providers, and us.

Kimberly George offers the following:

> Case managers can play critical roles in our achieving a positive outcome. It is often challenging for us to deal with an injury. Needing to deal with all the aspects of the "system" while we are injured can be overwhelming.
>
> Case managers will assist us in coordinating our care and connecting us with needed resources. They should be our advocates and help us define our expectations regarding our claims, medical treatments, and/or disabilities, as we may need. When we meet with case managers we should share our concerns and our goals. They will work with us in developing a case-management plan—but we must always stay actively involved.

Vocational Rehabilitation Counselors

Even with all possible accommodations we may face limitations or restrictions that won't allow us to return to our prior jobs. Then we need to find new jobs within our changed capabilities.

Vocational rehabilitation counselors develop and implement return-to-work plans. Effective vocational rehabilitation counselors evaluate our capabilities, interests, and skills and advise us on strategies to improve our capabilities and skills. Rehabilitation may involve our learning new skills or trades. These counselors will assist us in job searches and guide us in applying and interviewing for new jobs.

When employment is tight, and few jobs may be available, vocational rehabilitation may be less successful and employers and insurers may be less willing to support it.

If we were working and have been injured or ill, and cannot perform the functions of our old job the same as we did before, our first question for our employer can be "How will you now accommodate me to assist my successful return to my job?" If our employer is unable or unwilling to offer us accommodations that allow us to return to our old job, our next question can be "What other jobs will you offer me for which I have or may develop the needed capabilities?" If our employer is large enough to have different types of work options, we are more likely to be provided with offers falling within our capabilities.

Our employer may be unable or unwilling to offer us accommodations to either return to our old job or find worthwhile employment in a new job. Then we need to discuss with our claims adjuster or lawyer if vocational rehabilitation would be appropriate. Vocational rehabilitation counselors are required to help us return to work with our current employer if possible before guiding us toward alternative employment or retraining.

Independent Medical Evaluators

Medical evaluators often review personal injury, workers' compensation, or other disability claims. An independent medical evaluation (IME) is an assessment performed by a doctor not otherwise involved in our care. Doctors performing these evaluations may be certified by the American Academy of Disability Evaluating Physicians or the American Board of Independent Medical Examiners.

Independent medical evaluators may range from highly skilled and truly independent to those who are less skilled and with predetermined agendas.

Independent medical evaluations typically are requested and paid for by employers or insurers. They may also be obtained by lawyers representing us. Our relationship with an independent medical evaluator differs from that with our treating doctor. We will have no doctor/patient or therapist/patient relationship with our independent medical evaluator. We cannot expect independent medical evaluators to honor any confidences we might share with them. They do not have any professional obligations to us; their only professional obligations are to those who have hired them. Regardless of who is paying them for their time, evaluators are expected to base their opinions solely on the facts and current medical science.

Independent medical evaluations may be done to clarify or validate the cause of our problems—that is, are our problems caused by a specific injury?—or to provide an assessment on whether we are now as healthy as we are going to become. Evaluators may be asked to assess our residual impairment. Evaluations may be used to assess ability to return to work—to determine how disabled we may be. They may be used to assess the appropriateness of past and current healthcare and provide suggestions for future healthcare.

It should not surprise us when independent medical evaluators develop opinions different from those of our treating doctors. Reasonable doctors may disagree. Deciding which opinion is more correct involves assessing the accuracy and thoroughness of the data collected and the accuracy of the interpretations of these data.

If we are requested to undergo an evaluation we should be advised, well in advance, of the scheduled date and time and who our evaluator will be. Before the evaluation the evaluator ought to have obtained and reviewed our medical records so that they are knowledgeable about our case. At the evaluation we should expect the evaluator to obtain our complete medical history, perform a physical examination, and fully inform us about what testing and/or evaluations will occur.

After their evaluation the doctor will prepare and provide a report to their client. Again, as we will have no doctor/patient or therapist/patient relationship with our evaluator, we cannot expect to receive the report directly from this doctor. If our lawyers requested the evaluation, we have a right to review the document. Our claims adjuster or the defense lawyer may choose to provide us a copy of any evaluation they requested—but they are often not obligated to do so.

For our independent medical evaluation:
- We want to carefully review the credentials of the assigned evaluator *before* the scheduled evaluation and make sure the evaluator practices in an appropriate specialty.
- We should bring pertinent medical records and x-rays if we can readily access this documentation. These records *should* have been obtained and reviewed by the independent medical evaluator—but we cannot always count on this. It is to our benefit to have a thorough evaluation.
- We should show up on time and anticipate that the evaluation will take at least an hour—or longer if our problem is complex or includes a psychological evaluation.
- We should record the times for our entire evaluation process including our arrival, the start and end times of the interview, the

start and end times of the physical examination, and any possible delays in our being processed.

- We should consider having someone we trust accompany us to provide us emotional support and the benefit of another perspective. In many jurisdictions we will have the right to have someone accompany us. In other jurisdictions some independent medical evaluators, however, may not allow others to be present during our actual evaluation. If we have a lawyer, that individual or a representative may usually accompany us.
- We should always be courteous and respectful. If we become angry or act inappropriately, it is only natural our evaluator may react negatively.
- We should feel free to ask the evaluator to provide explanations for all tests and/or evaluations being performed.
- We should be honest and never exaggerate our symptoms. If we omit pertinent history or exaggerate our problems, our credibility will be damaged.
- We should be as cooperative as possible during our examination and fully demonstrate our capabilities. Inconsistencies in our responses are exactly what independent medical evaluators are trained to observe.
- Following our evaluation we should document what occurred.
- If we can get a copy of the evaluation, we should provide one for our treating doctors and request they review it. We want to check if the report is accurate and identify possible conflicts between the opinions of the evaluator and those of our treating doctors. Sometimes the evaluator may provide new insights into our condition.
- When we have serious concerns regarding the integrity of the evaluation we may request our own doctors perform similar examinations. If we have legal representation, we can ask our lawyers to secure their own evaluations.

We need to understand that independent medical evaluations are often an inescapable part of our claims and insurance and disability processes.

Employers—Our Jobs

Our employers provide us our jobs. In their evaluations of our ability to perform our jobs, our employers have significant say in whether or not we are "disabled."

We all hope we will work in healthy environments, perform jobs that are not excessively risky, have some degree of control over our immediate tasks, and have supportive co-workers and supervisors. Sometimes we will. But sometimes we won't.

Smart employers value their employees and care for them. Smart employers demonstrate their caring by providing their employees access to quality healthcare. If we face injury or illness, smart employers will be actively engaged in our staying at or quickly returning to our jobs. Unfortunately, not all of our employers will be smart.

If we face injury or illness we should expect our employers to seek information from our doctors about what tasks we can accomplish. If we face medical limitations (things we cannot do) or restrictions (things we should not do because they pose a risk to us or others), our employers need to make sure these are addressed. Smart employers value their employees and provide reasonable accommodations for injury or illness. Such accommodations may include modifications of activities, job focus, or work hours.

Employers are legally and morally responsible for maintaining a safe workplace and treating us fairly. When we are facing medical issues our employers have a responsibility to provide our doctors with necessary work-related information—including information on what activities, chemicals, or machinery may be involved in our jobs.

Employers must participate in workers' compensation insurance or be self-insured. All but the smallest of employers must honor legal mandates including holding our jobs for up to twelve weeks if we are injured or ill.

Employers in the United States must make reasonable accommodations for those of us otherwise qualified employees with disabilities as specified in the Americans with Disabilities Act. If we find it necessary to file an injury or illness medical claim, our employers need to cooperate with others—including the claims adjuster, healthcare providers, and legal representation—involved with processing our claim.

We should expect that it would be extremely rare for our doctors to say that we are unable to perform our job. Such an evaluation would be reasonable only if we have had a catastrophic problem (such as extensive paralysis) or we pose a risk to others (we become contagious or our impairments pose safety hazards for others) or ourselves (by being asked or required to perform tasks beyond our current capabilities).

In most cases we should expect our doctors to be able to provide specific information on what tasks we can and cannot perform. We must expect to provide this information to our employers and ask that they provide us reasonable accommodations to let us continue at our old jobs, if possible, or move to other worthwhile jobs, if necessary.

If our employers tell us they can no longer provide us a worthwhile job we need to ask why—and then we need to consider our most appropriate next steps.

Bob Steggert, former co-chair of the National Academy of Social Insurance's Workers' Compensation Steering Committee and retired vice president of casualty claims for Marriott International, offers the following concerning what we should expect from employers when we face a potentially disabling injury or illness:

> It's not surprising that many employers now refer to the once-traditional "boss-worker" employee relationship in ways acknowledging the key contributions modern "employees" make to the success of our companies. We are now more commonly recognized as "associates," "colleagues," "team members" or other terms more clearly addressing our contributions.
>
> This recognition that we employees form a key "asset" to the success of our employers is both powerful and profound. Informed employers must now seek to proactively address any injuries or illnesses we may face as employees so as to help with and support our optimal healthcare outcomes and speedy return-to-work productivity.
>
> This level of support requires the full attention of our employers (as opposed to their simply complying with regulatory reporting) when dealing with our injuries or illnesses. This attention must entail top-down enterprise leadership starting with the most senior management and/or owners. It requires effective and timely communications and good-faith coordination including all interested parties—especially *us*.
>
> Immediate problem resolutions, timely healthcare delivery and compensation, and optimal return-to-work coordination are essential.

In the United States virtually all employers have duties which cannot be delegated regarding honoring the requirements of the Americans with Disabilities Act (ADA) and the Family Medical Leave Act (FMLA). These laws often add to other contract and state-defined obligations concerning disability-claims management and return-to-work efforts.

Countless variables are involved in determining optimal outcomes. We should expect all interested parties—including ourselves—to stay focused on optimal end-goals and act entirely in good faith. At the same time, we need to be on the alert for and recognize possible "toxic" or other behaviors inconsistent with good faith in our efforts to reach our optimal end-goal.

Disability, sadly, is an occasional reality in human endeavors. Still, no matter the physical realities we face, we must strive for the optimal outcomes achievable in every situation and expect all parties to act with integrity and compassion. We deserve, and should accept, no less.

Internet—A Complex Web

Today the Internet will frequently be a significant resource in healthcare issues. In today's electronic society, when many of us (particularly the younger among us) have a question or need information, our first inclination may be to use an Internet search to seek answers.

While the Internet provides us overwhelmingly huge volumes of information on health and disability issues, this information has one massive problem—much of the medical information on the Internet is simply wrong and/or unreliable. Much of the information posted on the Internet is commercially biased or is little more than the unsubstantiated beliefs of an opinionated individual or group.

Often, because such sites may be generated by large and well-funded commercial enterprises, the most biased commercial sites will come up at the top of Internet searches. Meanwhile our more reliable, evidence-based, sites and information will be buried deep in the search results.

We have to search carefully for and validate "evidence-based" information. Even then, much of the "evidence-based" information we may find will be written by and for medical professionals and we may not be able to fully understand what is being said.

We are generally safe in our information search if we review medical-information sites ending in ".gov" run by the U.S. or other governments (such as the Australian site: http://www.health.gov. au/). Although many of us may have political issues with the U.S. or other governments under given administrations, generally government medical-information sites are maintained by medical professionals and provide scientifically reliable evidence-based information.

Medical-information sites generated by major medical schools (often ending in ".edu") or respected research hospitals will also generally be good sources for our research. As discussed earlier, the Cochrane Collaboration is a highly regarded resource for evidence-based medicine. A list of evidence-based medical websites may be found in the back of *Living Abled and Healthy* and is available at www.livingabled.com.

As we search the Internet for information on our health, medical, and/or disability concerns we want to consider each site we view with the following concerns:

- Who runs the site? Check the information shown in the "About Us" section of the site to determine who is controlling the postings. Even then, be suspicious, as many commercially funded sites will be posted with vague and not-obviously-commercial identifications.
- Why does this site exist and what is its purpose? If the site exists simply to offer information, it may still be accurate or inaccurate. However if the site exists primarily to sell a product or raise money we need to expect substantial bias in the information being presented.
- What is the original source of the information posted? Where does this information come from? Is it provided by reliable, unbiased, evidence-based sources?
- How is the information documented? Is it based on peer-reviewed, evidence-based scientific studies with accessible references to the underlying medical research?
- How has the information been reviewed and revised before being posted? Does the site provide information regarding the individuals reviewing and revising the information being posted and their medical or scientific credentials?

- How current is the information? When was the site last updated?
- What other sites does this site link to? Are these other sites highly reputable and unbiased or do the links lead to commercial and/or opinionated sites?
- What information does this site collect about visitors—us—and why?
- How does this site manage interactions with visitors?
- Can the accuracy of any information received via email be verified?
- Is the information being offered in chat rooms associated with this site accurate?

If the information we find on the Internet is accurate and evidence-based, this information may provide us a good basis for our informed decisions and may be valuable to us. On the other hand, if the information we find on the Internet is inaccurate and/or biased any decisions we make based upon such information may significantly harm us. We must never believe everything we read simply because it has been posted to the Internet.

Advocacy Groups—Doing Our Best?

Advocacy groups promoting greater attention to our specific health and medical concerns may provide us significant benefits. They often offer us connections to others experiencing similar problems. Many advocacy groups focus on increasing funding for evidence-based research and responses for concerns affecting us and those we care for. Such groups may use the Internet and multiple other forms of media and direct communications to increase public awareness of their cause and to influence public opinion on our behalf.

Sometimes, however, even our most well-intentioned advocacy groups may actually prove harmful—sometimes extremely harmful—to our health.

It all depends on who has organized our advocacy group, what their underlying motives may be, and the level and accuracy of knowledge generated and presented by the members of the advocacy group.

Advocacy groups are often based on a shared common concern with a specific health condition, illness, or type of injury. Frequently we will also have shared commercial, moral, political, or religious drivers for our advocacy groups. It is not unusual for the members of these groups to be fervent believers in the positions espoused by our group while the group leadership may be far more commercially focused.

We need to be attentive to the underlying drivers of advocacy groups with which we come into contact. As always, our first concern should be to see if the positions and/or solutions advocated are derived from evidence-based research.

There are advocacy groups where we may share a common belief system not supported by currently available evidence-based research. The positions and/or solutions we may advocate in such groups may be inaccurate and/or unhealthy and, sadly, we may be coming together and doing little more than reinforcing each other's problems.

We may become involved in an advocacy group promoted by a charismatic leader who gains personally, often financially, from the group recognition. This may be particularly common with advocacy groups sharing a common focus on symptoms when the best of contemporary evidence-based research is currently unable to identify any definitive evidence for our problems. Even when lacking any currently available evidence-based support for their beliefs, such advocacy groups (and those of us who may be supporting these groups) may become effective in swaying public opinion and shaping government and fiscal policy, if not scientific debate.

Advocacy groups may help us the most by generating and coordinating support groups for those of us facing shared problems—and often for those supporting us as we face our problems.

Many advocacy groups have highly commendable purposes supporting increased evidence-based research and responses. Others are less clear in their support of evidence-based medicine and, in the worst of cases, may actually be doing more harm than good.

Media—Reliable Sources?

Today's media—in the forms of blogs, books, Internet, magazines, movies, newspapers, radio, social media, and television—constantly bombard us with massive levels of information overload. Just like the Internet (as earlier discussed), the rest of our whole range of media choices provide us with a great deal of information—information which may, or may not, be accurate.

We must always be aware that all media strive, essentially, to gain more visibility. As with all other "life forms," media's first drive is for survival—and media survival means outside attention and, later if not sooner, some form of support.

As we draw our selected tiny stream of media intake from the vast flood of media flowing past us, we need to be attentive to the many forms of bias that may be hidden, or even not so hidden, in our media intake. Common biases to which we must always be attentive may include advertising, corporate sponsorship, political, and/or religious bias.

Sensationalism—often without regard for any particular bias—is an enormous issue with health and medical reporting. The more a health or medical issue may be hyped into a death-threat scare—or a life-saving miracle—the more likely it is to see intensive media attention.

New scientific findings, often presented in conservative and controlled fashions by their discoverers and the true scientific press, may be hyped into a massive immediate threat to life as we know it by popular media. Building upon an always-popular aphorism, we need to take all such news of dire impending disasters—or equally of life-saving new miracles—with much more than the traditional "grain of salt."

11

Diagnosing and Treating

I used to just trust everything my doctors told me.
Now I demand to know a lot more about any tests and
treatments my doctors recommend.
I take less medication now and actually feel better and
stronger.
Even nicer, my life is getting a lot simpler.

We should expect our healthcare providers to accurately diagnose our problems and then identify appropriate treatments. We must participate actively in all decisions about our care. Our healthcare providers should present us with recommended treatment plans that identify the expected benefits, a time frame for these expectations to be achieved, and the possible problems from these treatments.

SPICE

Alan Colledge, MD, conceived the "SPICE" approach for our medical problems. "SPICE" is an acronym for "Simplicity, Proximity, Immediacy, Centrality, and Expectancy." Colledge based his system on experience in caring for wounded military. It has since been applied to the management of workplace injuries. Possible applications for this system go far beyond both situations.

Simplicity reflects the belief that simple problems treated simply usually remain simple problems while simple problems treated in complex fashions often become complex problems. Military medical workers found that ominous diagnoses, complicated tests, and extensive treatment for minor problems generated or strengthened beliefs of wounded military in being seriously injured or ill. Our beliefs often lead to our chronic symptoms and disability.

Common problems, by definition, occur commonly. When we have a common problem, such as back pain, we need be aware that pain may serve as a "red flag" suggesting we may be facing something seriously wrong—such as cancer. We need to also recognize that, the vast majority of times, back pain is simply just normal common back pain and we will be best off treating the problem as simply as possible.

While many of us may become concerned our pain is caused by a serious problem, the reality is that few of us will have serious underlying problems or will find any benefit from extensive treatments or surgery. Far too often we get far too many tests and treatments.

Simplicity applies to diagnoses. We want diagnostic labeling to be as simple and straightforward as possible. Wrong or complex diagnoses can be devastating even without underlying causes. We will stay healthier when doctors provide us with accurate and simple diagnoses.

Simplicity applies to testing. While the vast majority of diagnoses are generated from our medical histories, sometimes we will need diagnostic testing. But testing is only valuable if the test results may affect our treatment.

James Andrews, a sports-medicine orthopedist in Gulf Breeze, Florida, wanted to test his suspicion that the results from expensive MRI scans might be misleading. He had the shoulders of thirty-one perfectly healthy professional baseball pitchers scanned. The pitchers were not injured and had no pain complaints. But Andrews' MRI scans found 90 percent of the scanned pitchers displayed abnormal shoulder cartilage and 87 percent of them displayed abnormal rotator-cuff tendons. He concluded, "If you want an excuse to operate on a pitcher's throwing shoulder, just get an MRI."

Simplicity applies to treatment. Treatment must be based on decisions supported by scientific evidence. This applies to all treatment, including injections, other medications, surgeries, and other therapies.

Proximity reflects allowing and encouraging us to remain engaged in normal everyday activities. When we are allowed and encouraged to continue everyday activities we are likely to heal faster.

Immediacy reflects the need for our problems to generally be treated as quickly as possible. Generally, promptly providing us any needed treatments will offer the best possible results. Occasionally, however, for some issues, the more prudent approach is to allow some waiting—often to see if our bodies may be able to successfully respond to our problems without outside interventions.

Centrality reflects the need for everyone involved in our treatment—including us—to have a common goal. Injuries may generate different or conflicting goals among the various participants in our treatment. Healthcare providers will usually share our goal of restoring health as simply and as quickly as possible. However, financial incentives for some healthcare providers to generate treatments, needed or not, are real—and may produce conflicted goals. Employers may or may not want us to return to our jobs. Lawyers may also be conflicted.

Expectancy reflects the concept that we will often fulfill the expectations we and others generate. Beliefs are powerful almost beyond our imaginations. When healthcare providers are optimistic and expect us to recover we will tend to absorb their expectations and attitudes and recover more quickly.

Drugs

When we see our doctors about medical problems many of us expect the visit will generate a drug prescription. We seek something tangible from visiting doctors. In the United States, our mindset regarding drugs as the way to cure every medical complaint is constantly reinforced by intensive drug advertising.

Among the so-called "developed" nations who have addressed this concern, only the United States and New Zealand allow drug companies to advertise directly to consumers—us. In the United States we are bombarded by drug commercials encouraging us to identify with others who have benefited from these drugs. The advertised call to action is "Ask your doctor if (Brand X) is right for you."

Doctors usually face busy, over-scheduled, time-restrained patient commitments. They may easily find it more time-efficient to write us a prescription than to spend time educating us.

We must require whatever time it takes for us to be fully informed about both our drug and non-drug treatment options. We need to be more discerning about what drugs we need—if we need any at all. Prescription drugs can be useful—for the right patient, the right condition, and at the right time. But we do not need many of the medications we are prescribed—and all medications involve some risk.

"Big Pharma"—The drug industry ("Big Pharma") is not just "big"— it is almost unimaginably huge. Legal drug manufacturing globally generates more than $950 billion in annual income. The United States provides almost a third of this—around $300 billion annually.

For every medical complaint, we and our doctors have to decide, will the benefits of taking a given drug exceed the cost and the risks of using that drug? We want treatments based on sound science and to believe our doctors are fully informed about any drug they might prescribe. This is not always true.

Drugs are almost always tested by the same companies who want to manufacture and sell them. Drugs are frequently tested in poorly designed clinical trials.

In his book *Bad Pharma,* British doctor Ben Goldacre concluded, "the whole edifice of medicine is broken" because evidence on drug treatments is distorted by the drug industry. Goldacre is not alone in his beliefs.

Marcia Angell, MD, was editor-in-chief of the renowned reference *The New England Journal of Medicine.* In that role she developed insights into the drug industry. Her book, *The Truth About the Drug Companies,* examines drug companies' shifting focus from discovering and manufacturing useful drugs to becoming vast marketing machines. She documents drug companies routinely relying on publicly funded institutions for their basic research, rigging clinical trials to make their products look better, stretching out government-granted exclusive marketing rights for years, and flooding the drug market with copycat drugs costing far more than the older, now patent-free, drugs they mimic but being no more effective.

Ray Strand, a family doctor, in *Death by Prescription,* noted that most U.S. doctors have minimal training in pharmacology and are not aware of the problems occurring with new drugs and drug interactions.

He believes we take far too many medications when we have better ways to manage our health.

John Abramson, MD, reveals, in *Overdosed America: The Broken Promise of American Medicine,* the ways in which drug companies compromise our health, mislead doctors, and misrepresent statistical evidence. The good news, he believes, is that scientific evidence demonstrates that reclaiming responsibility for our health can be more effective than our taking the newest drugs.

The drug industry significantly influences which healthcare problems are addressed, publicized, and researched. Big Pharma influences drug trials. The industry is deeply committed to marketing.

If we want to stay healthy we need to stay skeptical *every* time we are prescribed a drug.

Big Pharma=Really Big Marketing—Drug-industry advertising to doctors and to the public—us—is highly sophisticated. Promotional efforts include manipulating public media to promote certain diseases as needing drug treatment, paying doctors to support specific drugs at professional meetings, and targeting consumer-advocacy groups. These efforts are reinforced by lobbying and political contributions to influence government regulatory bodies.

Contemporary medical articles are now frequently generated by non-MD "ghostwriters," not identified as authors, who are paid by device manufacturers and drug companies which then solicit doctors to sign on as authors. A 2009 article in *The New York Times* estimated that 11 percent of *The New England Journal of Medicine* articles were written by ghostwriters.

Drug companies have proven that direct-to-consumer—us—advertising is extremely effective. Drug ads start by leading us to believe we have some condition for which the advertised drug is our best solution. Direct-to-consumer advertising is biased so as to lead us to demand from our doctors the medications we see advertised.

Doctor Knowledge—Clinical pharmacology studies how our medications are absorbed and eliminated, how they work, and what side effects they produce. Most U.S. medical schools require *no* formal courses in clinical pharmacology.

Doctors may be taught to prescribe certain drugs for certain conditions but they typically are not trained to know how these drugs are absorbed and metabolized in our bodies; how one drug interacts with other drugs or even with our common foods; or how our genetic differences alter our drug responses.

Pharmacists have more training in pharmacology than most doctors. Yet we rarely question our pharmacists while continuing to rely on doctors for drug information.

Off-Label Use—The U.S. Food and Drug Administration (FDA) regulates, to some degree, manufacturers' claims concerning each drug. Manufacturers are required to list the conditions for which their medications have been tested and approved. But doctors' legal prescription of drugs is not limited to only those tested and approved conditions. Doctors may legally prescribe drugs for conditions other than those listed by the manufacturer and approved by the Food and Drug Administration. This is "off-label" use.

Drug companies pay doctors to promote off-label uses of their drugs. One company paid for five thousand doctors to fly to and stay at Caribbean resorts where they were paid two-thousand dollar "honoraria" to listen to lectures about one drug (Bextra®) between their golf games and massages. Pfizer, the maker of Bextra®, later paid the U.S. government $1.3 billion in criminal fines related to the "off-label" marketing of Bextra®, a now-withdrawn pain medication.

When our doctor recommends an "off-label" use we want to question both the doctor and our pharmacist about the wisdom of this prescription—and its possible problems.

Side Effects and Risks—Journalist Melody Petersen estimated, in *Our Daily Meds: How the Pharmaceutical Companies Transformed Themselves Into Slick Marketing Machines and Hooked the Nation on Prescription Drugs,* that almost three times as many Americans die each year from prescription drugs than are being killed in car accidents.

This is approximately one hundred thousand Americans each year—a staggering 270 every day.

Deaths from prescription drug overdoses quadrupled from 1999 to 2010. Prescription drugs are now involved in more than half of all reported U.S. drug overdoses—in 2010 this meant 22,134 of the 38,329 reported drug-overdose deaths. Drugs from our nation's pharmacies are now killing more people than drugs from our nation's illegal labs and illegal international smugglers. The majority of prescription drug overdoses involved opioid pain medications such as oxycodone and morphine.

All medications are associated with side effects and risks—some rare and mild and some more common and possibly deadly. Side effects are the unintended consequences we may face from taking a drug. Many of us recognize that certain types of allergy drugs (antihistamines) may make us drowsy. This is a side effect.

Other common drug side effects include allergic reactions, bowel problems, heart palpitations, insomnia, muscle aches, and nausea and vomiting. Side effects may also produce even more serious problems including confusion, hallucinations, kidney damage, liver damage, memory loss, suicidal ideation, and others. Sometimes it may take years of large-scale use of a prescription medication for doctors to identify all of its significant side effects.

The more medications we take the more likely we are to suffer from drug interactions. Some interactions make drugs more or less effective for whatever reason we are taking them while others may increase the likelihood and/or severity of side effects.

Package Inserts—Prescription (and even non-prescription) medications always come with some documentation offering information about the medication. If we are honest, we will admit that most of us just ignore all the fine print (if we can even read it) and just look at the packaging. We really must try to do better than this.

Information that may be critical to us may be buried in that fine print. Often the information is written with such complex language we simply cannot understand all of it. But we should always try to read it anyway and look for key words we may have heard earlier from doctors or seen in other descriptions of our problems. When we see key words we know are important to us—even if we do not understand exactly what is being said—we should demand explanations from our doctors or pharmacists before agreeing to take these medications. While all of the documentation is important, we really want to try to at least scan, looking for recognizable key words, some of the most important sections:

- Highlights—The most important information about benefits and risks.
- Date of initial product approval—The longer a drug has been approved the greater our collective experience has been with this medication.
- Indications and usage—If the reason we are taking this medication is *not* listed then we are being prescribed this drug for an "off label" use—and we should demand to know why.
- Contraindications—These are the reasons we should *not* use this drug—and we always want to read this section. Pregnancy or other medical conditions are frequent contraindications.
- Warnings—We should review our possible serious side effects and weigh these against our potential benefits.
- Precautions—The steps we need to follow to take our medication safely.
- Overdose—What happens if we take too much and what to do about it. This information alone makes it useful to keep the documentation until we finish all the medication—just in case.
- Dosage and administration—We can check how much we were told to take against the official recommendation—number or dosage-size mistakes are easy in prescription processing.
- How supplied—This physical description of the medication can warn us if the medication we have been given is *not* the medication being described—mistakes happen in prescription processing.

Drug Risks versus Benefits—We want to approach all drugs, both prescription and over-the-counter, with skepticism. We need to be informed. Medications can help our health and recovery or they can hurt us—or, sometimes, both. We need to decide on our benefits versus our risks. We make risk/benefit decisions all the time in other aspects of our lives—we need to do this with our medications.

We should:

- Keep a list of the medications we take, both prescription and over-the-counter, and be able to share this list with our doctors and pharmacists.
- Avoid demanding specific medications from our doctors.
- Ask, when our doctor prescribes an unfamiliar medication:
    - What are my alternatives?
    - What are the common experiences with this drug?
    - Will this drug interact with my other medications?
    - What are the side effects and risks?
- Is this drug FDA approved for this use?
- Try to avoid new drugs unless we have serious or unusual conditions and the drug may be a scientifically documented medical "breakthrough."
- Try to avoid accepting drugs being dispensed from our doctors' offices. If we are offered drugs dispensed from our doctor's office we are entitled to ask how their prices compare to the prices of regular pharmacies and especially to those pharmacies of "big box" retailers (which often offer the lowest prices).
- Review the drug documentation and ask our doctor or pharmacist any questions we may have.
- Try to learn more online about our drugs from government or large medical school or respected research hospital websites and avoid relying on sites having a commercial bias. A list of evidence-based medical websites may be found in the back of *Living Abled and Healthy* and is available at www.livingabled.com.

If we are asked to participate in a drug trial we should require written evidence that the trial has been publicly registered.

With all of our treatments we need to become as knowledgeable as possible about our potential benefits and risks—and then make our informed decisions.

Opioids—Much of the Western world is currently experiencing an opioid epidemic. Inappropriate and excessive use of opioids destroys lives and often kills. It is well worth our time and effort to pay particular attention to possibly accepting prescriptions for opioids and other narcotics.

Opioids are among the world's oldest known drugs. They are chemicals that bind to opioid receptors in our nervous systems. Initially use of opioids will decrease our perception of pain and provide a sense of euphoria (intense happiness and self-confidence).

The body creates its own opioid-peptides known as endorphins. These chemicals are produced by the pituitary gland in the hypothalamus in the brain when we eat spicy food, endure pain, exercise, or are sexually active and achieve orgasm.

Strenuous exercise is particularly effective for generating these endorphins as they are released during long workouts of moderate or high intensity. Often described as our "runner's high," endorphin production also occurs with other forms of exercise as well.

The earliest known reference to opium poppy cultivation is from 3400 BCE. The Sumerians called opium poppies "hul gil," the "joy plant." In the ninth century BCE, Homer's *Odyssey* told how "Presently she cast a drug into the wine of which they drank to lull all pain and anger and bring forgetfulness of every sorry."

In 1804 morphine, the first active alkaloid extracted from the opium poppy plant, was isolated. In 1874 diacetylmorphine or diamorphine (known as heroin when manufactured and sold illegally) was synthesized from morphine and first sold by Bayer in 1898. Since the mid-1900s drug companies have developed numerous synthetic opioids.

Initially these synthetic opioids were developed and approved for treating end-stage-cancer pain. Doctors with patients—us—having other types of chronic pain began, with strong encouragement from drug companies, prescribing opioids for these other cases of chronic pain. Chronic pain is challenging for us to experience and for our doctors to treat. We should be especially attentive when our doctor prescribes an opioid for pain unless we have cancer or a sudden and severe problem (such as a recent surgery or major trauma). If we are or a close relative or friend is on opioids we should be concerned. Our risks may well exceed our benefits.

Risks of opioid use include addiction and adverse effects including death. Chronic opioid users may become physically and/or psychologically addicted. Stopping opioid medications may result in withdrawal symptoms. Common adverse reactions to opioids include constipation, drowsiness, dry mouth, itching, nausea and vomiting, and sexual dysfunction. Overdose results in decreased consciousness, slowing of the heart and breathing rates, and, in extreme cases, death. Medicaid populations are often at greater risk of opioid overdoses than non-Medicaid populations. Risks are increased when opioids are used along with alcohol, antidepressants, and/or tranquilizers.

There are many other concerns about opioids, including:

- Tolerance is likely. Over time the body adjusts to the medication and higher doses are required to produce the same effect.
- Opioid use may create a severe sensitivity to pain called hyperalgesia.
- With men, long-term use lowers testosterone resulting in osteoporosis and muscle weakness.

Epidemic opioid overuse in the United States is resulting in addiction and deaths:

- Since 2003, prescription opioids have been involved in more drug-overdose deaths than heroin or cocaine.
- Opioid overdoses killed 16,651 people in the United States in 2010. This is more than four times the 4,000 people who were killed by these drugs in 1999.
- In 2010, enough opioids were prescribed in the United States to medicate every American adult with a typical dose of 5 mg of hydrocodone (when combined with acetaminophen, often sold as Vicodin®) every four hours for three weeks.
- Most nonmedical users of prescription opioids get drugs which have been prescribed for others.
- A small percentage of U.S. doctors cause the majority of problems. Only 3 percent of U.S. doctors account for 62 percent of prescribed opioid pain relievers.
- Opioid abuse has been demonstrated in 9–41 percent of patients receiving chronic pain management.

Some doctors believe they are doing the right thing by prescribing pain relievers for us. And, for some of us, opioids may be appropriate if they reduce our pain and increase our function. Generally, especially with long-term use, opioids result in only modest reductions in our pain while creating significant risks. Risks are increased with:

- A history of alcohol, opioid, tobacco, or other substance abuse
- A history of chronic benzodiazepine (of which diazepam, trade named Valium®, may be the most recognized form) or other sedative use
- Personality disorders
- Depression and/or other psychological disorders
- A history of being away from our jobs for more than six months
- A history of a past poor response to opioids

What should we do if we are taking opioids or our doctor suggests we take opioids? We want to recognize that opioid treatment is associated with serious risks and many possible adverse reactions. Before beginning opioids we want to explore other approaches to dealing with chronic pain. We may have safer alternative medications including non-narcotic analgesics (such as acetaminophen), nonsteroidal anti-inflammatories (such as ibuprofen or naproxen), antineuropathic agents, and antidepressants. Antineuropathic pain medications are used to reduce nerve activity and pain hypersensitivity associated with conditions such as shingles, diabetic nerve pain, and certain other nerve disorders. Antidepressants are often helpful in reducing chronic pain, assisting with sleep, and improving function. We may find exercise or techniques such as cognitive behavioral therapy useful for pain relief.

If we determine we would benefit from prescription opioids we should use them as briefly as possible. We should ask our doctors what clinical guidelines they follow for opioid use. There are excellent guidelines, such as the "Guidelines for the Chronic Use of Opioids" by the American College of Occupational and Environmental Medicine, available for our doctors.

We should expect our doctors to first do a careful evaluation of pain complaints, obtain a comprehensive medical history, do a thorough physical examination, document functional difficulties, and generate appropriate physical and psychological evaluation reports. They need to discuss with us the potential benefits versus risks of opioid treatment.

We should expect them to use a treatment agreement documenting our understanding and expectations.

We should expect follow-up visits checking for adverse reactions and changes in functional abilities. We should expect we will be helped to discontinue opioid use as quickly as possible.

Doctor-Abetted Opioid Abuse—The majority of U.S. opioid prescriptions are generated by a small percentage of doctors. A still smaller percentage of doctors become operators of prescription-opioid "pill mills" selling tremendous quantities of prescription pain medications at great profit. But even a tiny number of extremely high-volume prescribers can drive the use of opioids, and of opioid addictions and overdose deaths, within a state and even in nearby states.

"Pill mills" identified as pain clinics provide large quantities of opioids to addicts and dealers without adequate, if any, medical cause, evaluations, or follow-up. Their "patients" are often addicts involved in illegal sales and distribution (called diversion) of the opiates. Pain clinics selling large quantities of prescription medications have been reported in Florida and Texas and probably exist elsewhere as well.

Doctor Dispensing—Tammie was waiting in her car in a parking lot when she was suddenly jolted at the same instant as she heard the crash. Her small car had just been struck in the rear by a much heavier Ford F-150 pickup. The driver of the truck was a teenage boy.

Oblivious to Tammie's car behind him, and with Tammie watching him in her mirror the entire time, he had backed right into her vehicle. Tammie's nerves were certainly rattled and she was not sure if she had any other problems.

Tammie was relieved to find that, other than deep scratches and some scuff marks on the bumper, her year-old Toyota Corolla appeared OK.

Tammie was thirty-seven and had never faced any significant health issues. She took no regular medications. She hoped she had not been hurt.

Tammie and the other driver exchanged insurance information. She knew her state mandated that minor vehicle accidents be handled as "no-fault" claims. She drove home, not feeling any immediate need to see a doctor.

The next morning Tammie knew her neck was stiff. She mentioned the accident to her friend Jane. Jane suggested Tammie was suffering from "whiplash," the same condition Jane had faced a year earlier and one that continued to cause her problems. Jane recommended that Tammie see Dr. Johnson at the Trauma Recovery Center—Johnson was the doctor a lawyer friend had recommended to Jane.

Dr. Johnson was able to see Tammie the same day. He confirmed the diagnosis of whiplash. He advised Tammie that whiplash could take months to heal and might even leave her with continuing problems. Since Tammie had actually helplessly watched the accident happening, Dr. Johnson also worried that Tammie might develop a post-traumatic stress disorder. Dr. Johnson made arrangements for Tammie to be treated three days a week with in-house physical and massage therapy services at his personally owned Trauma Recovery Center.

Dr. Johnson prescribed Tammie several medications and conveniently dispensed them right from his office. He told Tammie he would take care of billing her insurance company. Dr. Johnson prescribed Tammie two non-steroidal anti-inflammatories to help her pain, a muscle relaxer, and, to reduce the stomach upset often associated with the anti-inflammatories, a drug compound to inhibit gastric-acid secretion. Dr. Johnson reassured Tammie that if her pain did not stop quickly he would prescribe her stronger opioid pain relievers.

This was the first time Tammie had ever gotten medications directly from a doctor's office. However it was convenient to avoid the drugstore and she just assumed this was standard for accident victims. She was surprised she needed so many different medications but her doctor appeared sincerely concerned with her well-being.

Two weeks after Tammie's visit with Dr. Johnson her insurance company received a bill from a third-party billing organization. The bill showed Tammie had been prescribed diclofenac (a non-steroidal anti-inflammatory drug—"NSAID") for $200.74, naproxen (another NSAID) for $188.16, carisoprodol (a muscle relaxer) for $277.47, and omeprazole *(to reduce stomach problems often associated with NSAIDs) for $367.11, totaling $1,033.48.*

Tammie never saw the bill. Tammie also never knew the average total pharmacy price for her drugs would have been $261.16. Nor would she ever learn Dr. Johnson's actual cost for her medications was only $33.42.

To save his office the effort of billing, Dr. Johnson had sold Tammie's bill to a medical billing company for 70 percent—$723.44—of what the billing company charged Tammie's insurance. Dr. Johnson's profit on Tammie's drugs was $690.02 for her one-month supply. The longer Tammie takes to recover, the more Dr. Johnson profits by supplying Tammie's medications.

If Dr. Johnson has two hundred patients at his Trauma Recovery Center needing similar or more drugs each month, these prescriptions— without any billings for the care by Dr. Johnson or for physical- and massage-therapy sessions—would generate his Trauma Recovery Center an annual profit of over $1.65 million dollars.

How do we know what treatment is right? Evidence-based medical treatment guidelines serve as standards to determine if treatments are "reasonable, appropriate, and necessary." By such treatment guidelines, and in the opinions of most doctors, the medications Dr. Johnson prescribed Tammie were unreasonable, inappropriate, and unnecessary—but how was Tammie to know?

Tammie's problem was "whiplash," a strain to her neck muscles. Given the small level of collision forces involved, as evidenced by the minimal damage to her car, Tammie could be expected to recover quickly without medical attention.

Tammy received four prescriptions—two prescription non-steroidal anti-inflammatory drugs, the muscle-relaxer carisoprodol, and the gastric-acid-secretion inhibitor omeprazole. She did not need any of them. By most accepted medical standards Tammie needed only a mild non-prescription over-the-counter pain reliever like acetaminophen (commonly sold as Tylenol®). Acetaminophen is typically the preferred initial choice for treatment of acute pain.

With multiple drugs there is an increased risk of side effects and of drug interactions. Aside from cost issues, one difference between drugs dispensed from a doctor's office and drugs dispensed from a pharmacy is that when drugs are dispensed from a pharmacy—particularly from our regular pharmacy where we get all of our other drugs—there is a greater chance any potential drug interactions will be recognized.

Doctor dispensing has an extensive history up until about a hundred years ago. Doctor dispensing largely ended as retail pharmacies developed and became the primary sources for medications. Both state and federal drug-dispensing requirements multiplied and, arguably the most significant change, the number of available medications increased so greatly it became difficult for any doctor to stock a full inventory.

Today, doctor-dispensed medications are not usually about our benefits of speed and convenience—they are usually about our doctors making money. Even when we do not directly pay for our medications, ultimately we all do pay—inflated charges are reflected in our insurance premiums and taxes.

Interventional Pain Management

Interventional pain management uses injections and other treatments to reduce pain. Sometimes these may be helpful; other times they are not. Therapeutic injections are a significant source of revenue for some doctors and this may influence their decision to provide this treatment. We want to be sure the reasons given for providing these treatments are consistent with evidence-based medicine. Typically spinal blocks are done for specific indications and only after appropriate evaluation and alternative therapies have been tried. Most therapeutic injections address only symptoms and do nothing to resolve the underlying problem.

Surgery

Some surgery may be absolutely critical to our well-being. Other surgery may not. Again, everything depends on our specific situation.

As with any other treatment, the first step should be determining our problem. Unless we have sudden and severe problems such as airway blockages, severe broken bones, serious burns, major cuts with extensive bleeding, major internal-organ damage or internal bleeding, massive and spreading infection, or other equally serious problems, most surgical operations will be "elective." Elective surgeries are those we can choose to do or not to do—and we may take time to consider our decisions.

Generally we will always want to first explore non-surgical medical responses. If our condition offers no reasonable non-surgical alternatives or if we try non-surgical alternatives and we do not improve, and evidence-based medicine supports surgical intervention, then we may seriously consider surgery.

We want to always remember the old saying how "If our only tool is a hammer, we will treat everything as if it were a nail." This is especially true when using the hammer provides income to its user. When we consult surgeons about our concerns we need to expect they may believe surgery will be the best answer—this is what they know and the treatment for which they are paid.

When we consider surgery and what benefits we may gain from successful surgery we must also consider the risks we face from any surgery. Along with possible complications even from successful surgeries—such as post-operative infections and internal scarring—any surgery involving general anesthesia involves a small but real risk of death simply from the anesthesia.

When doctors recommend elective surgery it will almost always be worthwhile to secure a second opinion from another doctor—one having no relationship with our first doctor. If the opinions are different, we may wish to seek out a third opinion to see if we may find some consensus.

We must be careful to choose the most skillful doctor for any surgeries—typically this will be one who has done the specific procedure many times. For example, if we had carpal tunnel syndrome, usually we would want to have any surgery done by a hand surgeon rather than a general surgeon.

It may also be helpful to seek opinions from doctors practicing in different specialties. They will view the same problem from different perspectives benefitting from different experiences. For example, physical medicine and rehabilitation doctors may offer different perspectives from those of spinal surgeons.

Medical Devices

Doctors may use or recommend various medical devices. A medical device is any apparatus, implant, instrument, or other similar article intended for the diagnosis or treatment of disease. Medical devices range from simple wooden tongue depressors to complex programmable devices with microchip computer technology.

Unlike drugs, medical devices act through electrical, mechanical, physical, or thermal processes. Like drugs, medical devices may offer us great benefits—or they may not—and sometimes they may harm us.

Medical devices prescribed for treatments are not always as beneficial or as safe as advertised. Even with the best of manufacturers' intentions, huge numbers of medical devices—including artificial hips, heart stents, and pacemakers—have been recalled. The worst of these recalls involved devices surgically implanted, often with significant risk and substantial pain, within us.

When doctors prescribe medical devices we want to question why we need them—particularly if they do this on our first visit and dispense the devices from their offices. Prescribed devices may be as simple as back braces or "therapeutic" pillows or as complex as drug pumps or spinal-cord stimulators. We should carefully examine our problems and situations and consider whether evidence-based medicine supports such devices.

As discussed above concerning doctor-dispensed drugs, we want to be attentive to possible conflicts should our doctors prescribe medical devices they sell directly or in which they have financial interest.

When we face uncertainty, as we usually will, and the device doesn't involve surgery, trial testing would be completely appropriate. We should do our best to try to separate any real improvement in functioning or any real decrease in our pain from the likely placebo effect.

When we face uncertainty using a surgically implanted device we should be particularly careful. Many surgically implanted devices take us down one-way streets of non-reversible changes to our bodies.

We will never have complete certainty for any decisions—and many operations involving medical devices can offer us tremendous benefits—but the decision to surgically implant medical devices should always be made with great care.

Assistive Technology

Assistive (including adaptive and rehabilitative) technology refers to devices used by those of us with or without disabilities to achieve greater independence. Assistive technology includes any hardware, software, or other products that help us maintain or improve our functional capabilities.

Contemporary science has made amazing improvements in hardware and software helping us reduce the gap between impairment and disability. Amputated arms, hands, and legs are being replaced by more and more sophisticated prosthetics—the newest of these offering sophisticated technology substantially restoring function. There are new designs for devices increasing mobility such as braces, walkers, and wheelchairs (manual and powered). Communications may be enhanced both by low technology, such as communication boards made with cardboard or fuzzy felt, and high technology, such as screen readers and communications systems.

If we are dealing with significant impairment issues we want to explore assistive technology and how this may help us. We may wish to review the website for the Assistive Technology Industry Association (www.atia.org) as one possible starting point.

What Do We Do?

We need to always stay in control of our health and our healthcare. Doctors need to respect us as people—or we should find new doctors. Providers need to demonstrate compassion concerning our symptoms and convey interest in helping us evaluate and manage our problems. We should insist on evidence-based, functionally oriented treatment for identified physical, psychological, or psychiatric disorders.

Our first objective must be staying empowered and taking an active role in managing our health. Approaching our treatments with this attitude increases our control and reduces our suffering. It improves our coping with symptoms and achieving maximal function. While complete cures may not be possible with today's medical knowledge, our goal for any treatment must be to maximize function and control, if not cure, symptoms.

We should be reassured when diagnoses of common and treatable, and possibly less common and possibly untreatable, conditions have been ruled out. Doctors need to know when to stop testing and/or stop ineffective treatments. Sometimes ordering unending tests and multiple referrals to specialists for unexplained problems only increases our fears of possible mystery ailments.

Providers need to consider possible psychological or psychiatric disorders (especially personality disorders or depression)—even when we may not be receptive to hearing about such concerns. These disorders can coexist with physical problems. Our providers should consider possible problems with anger, manipulation, or motivation—again, even when we may not be receptive to hearing about such concerns.

Some healthcare providers must strengthen their resolve to "first do no harm." Their primary aim must always be to help us focus on improving function and reducing risk.

We should expect collaboration among all of our healthcare providers and a common understanding of the biopsychosocial approach.

Our healthcare providers must involve us in our treatments by helping us establish goals and encouraging our continuing participation in our favorite activities and our jobs.

12

What Next?

*Demanding information at every step of my medical
process has opened a new world for me.
I've learned to chart my own course, avoid allowing
others to take advantage of me and my situations, and
how to get to where I need to be.
Now I have to do what I can to share these new
understandings.*

Living Abled and Healthy has offered some principles for recovering
from injury or illness:
- Taking control of our life and health
- Staying positive
- Partnering with quality healthcare providers who practice
  evidence-based and data-driven medicine
- Approaching problems from a "biopsychosocial" perspective
- Weighing the risks and benefits of testing and treatment
- Focusing on a healthy body, mind, and spirit
- Choosing smart lifestyles including exercise, diet, and health
  habits
- Weighing the risks and benefits of involving lawyers
- Cooperating with other healthcare participants and avoiding
  unnecessary conflict
- Continuing with our jobs, if at all possible

These principles work only if we use them—and use them consistently.
If we do, we will more likely experience healthy and happy lives. We

179

can't stop our aging but good health can slow many debilitating changes and offer us a better quality of life.

Beyond examining what each of us can do personally about our own injury, illness, or disability issues, as *Living Abled and Healthy: Your Guide to Injury and Illness Recovery* just has, we need to ask ourselves what we can do about these issues as a society. Just as personal strengths and weaknesses often begin in childhood, collective social strengths and weaknesses shaping societies and nations are rooted decades before breaking the surface and becoming obvious.

Core solutions to social problems will not come from medicine; they will be reflections of the changes each of us must help make in cultures and social policies.

We need well-defined care and recovery plans for injuries and illnesses founded on evidence-based medicine. We need an effective flow of accurate information among employers, healthcare providers, insurers, and ourselves. We all need to work together to achieve our goal—experiencing healthy and happy lives.

We must avoid needlessly identifying ourselves—or allowing others to needlessly identify us—as injured, ill, or disabled. As long as casual acceptance of needless disability remains socially acceptable, more and more of us will be identified as disabled.

We must change health and disability systems—and the combined business, government, insurance, legal, and medical complexes driving these systems. At the moment, within the United States, certain health maintenance organizations (HMOs) appear to be addressing many of the issues noted earlier. It would be good if we could see many of the established and beneficial policies developed by the best of these health maintenance organizations adopted more broadly within the medical establishment. We need different systems of rewards for all participants so we will share a focus on health and function rather than on procedures and disability. Whenever we can we want to continue our activities and stay at our jobs.

We start our journey by believing in ourselves and our purpose. We embrace whatever challenges we face. We take control of our lives!

Acknowledgments

Words cannot express my joy in thanking my wife Cathy for her love, care, and support. I am especially appreciative of all of my family— my children Mindy, Allison, and Gina; my brothers Martin and Neil; and my parents Jean and Ken. They have provided me with wonderful learning experiences and improved my understanding of what life is all about. Thanks to my relatives and friends who, throughout the years, have encouraged and strengthened me.

I have much gratitude for my co-author, Henry Bennett, who made *Living Abled and Healthy: Your Guide to Injury and Illness Recovery* a reality. He contributed substantially to the shaping and presentation of this work and added new perspectives and information and transformed my vision and thoughts into our book.

Throughout my life I have benefited from countless individuals and groups who provided insights and inspiration. Colleagues and friends helped formulate the ideas and shared the information reflected in *Living Abled and Healthy*. I am deeply appreciative of them and how they have touched my life.

Special thanks is given to my contributors Robert Aurbach, JD; David DePaolo, JD; Kimberly George; Les Kertay, PhD; Norma Leclair, PhD; Steve Leclair, PhD; Preston H. Long, PhD, DC; Jon Seymour, MD; Bob Steggert; and Jaco Van Delden, PT. Their insights and friendships are deeply appreciated.

Many of my colleagues and others have nurtured my understanding of these issues and provided constructive feedback. It would be impossible to identify all of those who have provided guidance and encouragement over the years and those who have provided feedback on the manuscript. In particular I want to thank Lani Abrigana; George Azsoth; Steven Babitsky, JD; Kit Beuret; Lei Brady; Francis Brewer, DC; Lee Brown, RN; Ken Burtness; David Butts; Jennifer Christian, MD; Marianne Cloeren, MD; Alan Colledge, MD; Gary Cox, RN; Stephen

Demeter, MD, MPH; Anne Deschene; Lorne K. Direnfeld, MD; John Endicott, MD; John Enright; Lee H. Ensalada, MD, MPH; Julie Gilbert; William Gilmour; Marcos Iglesias, MD, MMM; Todd Ingram, JD; Steve Katz; Chuck Kelley, MD, MPH, MBA; Kimberly Lund, DO; Eileen Marx; Paul McNaughton; Kent Peterson, MD; William Pipkin, JD; Sili G. Raab; Henry Roth, MD; Ian B. Scott; Michael Sheppard, DC; Mora Stanley; James Talmage, MD; David Torrey, JD; Craig Uejo, MD, MPH; John Valente, JD; Averyl Wallis; and Pamela Warren, PhD. There are so many more people who have positively influenced my life; thank you.

Thanks to Marlin Ouverson of External Design for his creativity and vision. His superb website-development work is greatly appreciated. And thanks as well to Buzz and Jodi Belknap for developing electronic production files, Mary Harper for indexing, and Powell Berger for proofreading.

I truly appreciate the inspiration provided by Lou Darnell, Gregory Gadson, Bethany Hamilton, Craig MacFarlane, Victor Marx, Mile Stojkoski, Caroline Sylva, Nick Vujicic, the Wounded Warrior Amputee Softball Team, and innumerable others who, despite challenges, have demonstrated the ability to live joyful and productive lives.

I appreciate the insights and support provided by members of the First Presbyterian Church of Honolulu and my colleagues with the Praxis Partners Consortium.

Christopher R. Brigham   Oʻahu, 2014

❦ ❦ ❦

I would like to acknowledge the creativity and efforts of the lead author, Dr. Christopher R. Brigham, for whom this work is the product of both a lengthy and honored professional career and decades of attention to the concerns addressed. It has been a privilege to work on this publication.

I would also like to express my appreciation to the many colleagues who helped mentor and shape my professional efforts over decades. Without the opportunities provided and experience gained I would have been far less prepared to assist Dr. Brigham in bringing this work to the broad audience it will benefit.

Henry Bennett   Oʻahu, 2014

Resources

Internet Resources

Quality of the health information found on the Internet varies greatly. The following *free* websites are highly regarded within the medical community and are widely used to identify useful clinical information.

Commercial websites may also provide valuable clinical information with a paid subscription or on a fee-for-use basis.

Visit http://www.livingabled.com for current links.

Free Evidence-based Medicine and Treatment/ Practice Guidelines
- The Cochrane Collaboration—http://www.cochrane.org/
- Informed Medical Decisions Foundation—http://www. informedmedicaldecisions.org/
- MDGuidelines—http://www.mdguidelines.com/
- National Guideline Clearinghouse—http://www.guideline.gov/

Free Health Information
- MedlinePlus—http://www.nlm.nih.gov/medlineplus/
- Medscape—http://www.medscape.com/
- Merck Manuals—http://www.merckmanuals.com/
- UpToDate—http://www.uptodate.com/home/patient-search-widget/
- WebMD—http://www.webmd.com/

Free Medical Literature
- Educus—http://www.educus.com/
- PubMed—http://www.ncbi.nlm.nih.gov/pubmed/

Free and Useful Resources

- *ACPA Resource Guide to Chronic Pain Medications and Treatment*— http://www.theacpa.org/Consumer-Guide
- Body Mass Index Calculator—http://www.cdc.gov/healthyweight/assessing/bmi/adult_bmi/english_bmi_calculator/bmi_calculator.html
- Choosing a Doctor or Healthcare Service—http://www.nlm.nih.gov/medlineplus/choosingadoctororhealthcareservice.html
- Pain Management—http://www.swedish.org/media-files/documents/pain-and-headache-center/stomp-booklet.aspx
- State Workers' Compensation Officials posted by U.S. Department of Labor—http://www.dol.gov/owcp/dfec/regs/compliance/wc.htm

Forms

The website http://www.livingabled.com offers readers of *Living Abled and Healthy* extensive resources including many forms conveniently formatted for 8 ½"x 11" printing and numerous links to other resources and tools. These web-based resources are frequently updated to provide the most current information.

Bibliography

*Primary references are indicated with authors' names in **bold**.*
Visit http://www.livingabled.com/ability-health-resources/
bibliography/ for these and more hyperlinked references.

Abramson, J. 2005. *Overdosed America: The Broken Promise of American Medicine*. New York: Harper Perennial.

Alcabes, P. 2009. *Dread: How Fear and Fantasy Have Fueled Epidemics From the Black Death to Avian Flu*. New York: PublicAffairs.

Angell, M. 2004. *The Truth About the Drug Companies: How They Deceive Us and What to Do About It*. New York: Random House.

Bailey, E. 2011. *The Patient's Checklist: 10 Simple Hospital Checklists to Keep You Safe, Sane and Organized*. New York: Sterling.

Barsky, A.J., and **E.C. Deans.** 2006. *Stop Being Your Symptoms and Start Being Yourself*. New York: Collins.

Baur, S. 1988. *Hypochondria: Woeful Imaginings*. Berkeley, CA: University of California Press.

Bausell, R.B. 2007. *Snake Oil Science: The Truth About Complementary and Alternative Medicine*. New York: Oxford University Press.

Black, C.M. 2008. *Working For a Healthier Tomorrow*. London: The Stationery Office.

Bortz, W.M. 2011. *Next Medicine: The Science and Civics of Health*. New York: Oxford University Press.

Brawley, O.W. 2011. *How We Do Harm: A Doctor Breaks Ranks About Being Sick in America*. New York: St. Martin's Griffin.

Brownlee, S. 2007. *Overtreated: Why Too Much Medicine is Making Us Sicker and Poorer*. New York: Bloomsbury.

Cantor, C., with B.A. Fallon. 1996. *Phantom Illness: Shattering the Myth of Hypochondria*. Boston: Houghton Mifflin Company.

Carlat, D. 2010. *Unhinged: The Trouble with Psychiatry—A Doctor's Revelations About a Profession in Crisis*. New York: Free Press.

Cohen, E. 2010. *The Empowered Patient: How to Get the Right Diagnosis, Buy the Cheapest Drugs, Beat Your Insurance Company, and Get the Best Medical Care Every Time*. New York: Ballantine Books Trade Paperbacks.

Conrad, P. 2007. *The Medicalization of Society: On the Transformation of Human Conditions into Treatable Disorders*. Baltimore, MD: Johns Hopkins University Press.

Coulter, A. 2011. *Engaging Patients in Health Care*. Maidenhead, Berkshire, UK: Open University Press.

Deyo, R.A., and D.L. Patrick. 2005. *Hope or Hype: The Obsession with Medical Advances and the High Cost of False Promises*. New York: AMACOM.

Dineen, T. 2001. *Manufacturing Victims: What the Psychology Industry is Doing to People*. Third Edition. Montreal: Robert Davies Multimedia.

Doidge, N. 2007. *The Brain That Changes Itself: Stories of Personal Triumph from the Frontiers of Brain Science*. New York: Penguin Books.

Donoghue, P.J., and **M.E. Siegel.** 2000. *Sick and Tired of Feeling Sick and Tired: Living with Invisible Chronic Illness*. New Edition. New York: W.W. Norton.

Dossey, L. 1996. *Prayer Is Good Medicine: How to Reap the Healing Benefits of Prayer*. San Francisco: HarperSanFrancisco.

Dossey, L. 1999. *Reinventing Medicine: Beyond Mind-Body to a New Era of Healing*. San Francisco: HarperSanFrancisco.

Dyer, W.W. 2007. *Change Your Thoughts—Change Your Life*. Carlsbad, CA: Hay House.

Edwards, A., and G. Elwyn. 2009. *Shared Decision-Making in Health Care: Achieving Evidence-Based Patient Choice*. Second Edition. New York: Oxford University Press.

Elliott, C. 2010. *White Coat, Black Hat: Adventures on the Dark Side of Medicine.* Boston: Beacon.

Feinberg, S., with M. Leong, J. Christian, C. Pasero, A. Fong, and R. Feinberg. 2014. *ACPA Resource Guide to Chronic Pain Medication and Treatment.* Rocklin, CA: American Chronic Pain Association.

Foreman, J. 2014. *A Nation in Pain: Healing Our Biggest Health Problem.* New York: Oxford University Press.

Fox, M.J. 2009. *Always Looking Up: The Adventures of an Incurable Optimist.* New York: Hyperion.

Frances, A. 2013. *Saving Normal: An Insider's Revolt Against Out-of-Control Psychiatric Diagnosis, DSM-5, Big Pharma, and the Medicalization of Ordinary Life.* New York: William Morrow.

Geyman, J. 2008. *The Corrosion of Medicine: Can the Profession Reclaim Its Moral Legacy?* Monroe, MA: Common Courage.

Gibson, R., and **J.P. Singh.** 2010. *The Treatment Trap: How the Overuse of Medical Care is Wrecking Your Health and What You Can Do to Prevent It.* Chicago: Ivan R. Dee.

Goldacre, B. 2010. *Bad Science: Quacks, Hacks, and Big Pharma Flacks.* Reprint edition. New York: Faber and Faber.

Goldacre, B. 2013. *Bad Pharma: How Drug Companies Mislead Doctors and Harm Patients.* New York: Faber and Faber.

Greenberger, D., and C. Padesky. 1995. *Mind Over Mood: Change How You Feel by Changing the Way You Think.* New York: Guilford.

Groopman, J. 2005. *The Anatomy of Hope: How People Prevail in the Face of Illness.* Reprint edition. New York: Random House Trade Paperbacks.

Groopman, J. 2007. *How Doctors Think.* New York: Houghton Mifflin Company.

Groopman, J., and **P. Hartband.** 2011. *Your Medical Mind: How to Decide What is Right For You.* New York: Penguin Books.

Hadler, N.M. 2004. *The Last Well Person: How to Stay Well Despite the Health-Care System.* Montreal: McGill-Queen's University Press.

Hadler, N.M. 2008. *Worried Sick: A Prescription for Health in an Overtreated America.* Chapel Hill, NC: University of North Carolina Press.

Hadler, N.M. 2009. *Stabbed in the Back: Confronting Back Pain in an Overtreated Society*. Chapel Hill, NC: University of North Carolina Press.

Hadler, N.M. 2011. *Rethinking Aging: Growing Old and Living Well in an Overtreated Society*. Chapel Hill, NC: University of North Carolina Press.

Hadler, N.M. 2013. *The Citizen Patient: Reforming Health Care for the Sake of the Patient, Not the System*. Chapel Hill, NC: University of North Carolina Press.

Halligan, P.W., and M. Aylward, eds. 2006. *Power of Belief: Psychosocial Influence on Illness, Disability, and Medicine*. Oxford, UK: Oxford University Press.

Hanscom, D. 2012. *Back in Control: A Spine Surgeon's Roadmap Out of Chronic Pain*. Seattle: Vertus.

Helge, D. 1998. *Transforming Pain Into Power: Making the Most of Your Emotions*. Ontario, OR: Shimoda.

Horwitz, A.V. 2002. *Creating Mental Illness*. Chicago: University of Chicago Press.

Howard, P.K. 1994. *The Death of Common Sense: How Law is Suffocating America*. New York: Warner Books.

Howard, P.K. 2001. *The Collapse of the Common Good: How America's Lawsuit Culture Undermines Our Freedom*. New York: Ballantine.

Howard, P.K. 2009. *Life Without Lawyers: Liberating Americans From Too Much Law*. New York: W.W. Norton.

Hughes, R. 1993. *Culture of Complaint: The Fraying of America*. New York: The New York Public Library and Oxford University Press.

Illich, I. 2002. *Limits to Medicine: Medical Nemesis—The Expropriation of Health*. London: Marion Boyars.

Illich, I., I.K. Zola, J. McKnight, J. Caplan, and H. Shaiken. 2010. *Disabling Professions*. London: Marion Boyars.

Johnson, S.K. 2008. *Medically Unexplained Illness: Gender and Biopsychosocial Implications*. Washington, DC: American Psychological Association.

Justice, B. 2000. *Who Gets Sick: How Beliefs, Moods, and Thoughts Affect Your Health*. Second edition. Houston, TX: Peak.

Kaminer, W. 1993. *I'm Dysfunctional, You're Dysfunctional: The Recovery Movement and Other Self-Help Fashions.* New York: Vintage.

Kassirer, J.P. 2005. *On the Take: How Medicine's Complicity with Big Business Can Endanger Your Life.* New York: Oxford University Press.

Kent, D., and K.A. Quinlan. 1996. *Extraordinary People With Disabilities.* New York: Children's Press.

Lane, C. 2007. *Shyness: How Normal Behavior Became a Sickness.* New Haven, CT: Yale University Press.

Law, J. 2006. *Big Pharma: Exposing the Global Healthcare Agenda.* New York: Carroll and Graf.

Long, P. 2002. *The Naked Chiropractor: Insider's Guide to Combating Quackery and Winning the War Against Pain.* Tempe, AZ: Evidence-Based Health Services.

Long, P. 2013. *Chiropractic Abuse: An Insider's Lament.* New York: American Council on Science and Health.

Luskin, F. 2002. *Forgive for Good: A Proven Prescription for Health and Happiness.* New York: HarperCollins.

Luskin, F., and K.R. Pelletier. 2005. *Stress Free for Good: 10 Scientifically Proven Life Skills for Health and Happiness.* San Francisco: HarperSanFrancisco.

Mahar, M. 2006. *Money-Driven Medicine: The Real Reason Health Care Costs So Much.* New York: Collins.

Makary, M. 2012. *Unaccountable: What Hospitals Won't Tell You and How Transparency Can Revolutionize Health Care.* New York: Bloomsbury.

Malleson, A. 2002. *Whiplash and Other Useful Illnesses.* Montreal: McGill-Queen's University Press.

Manu, P., ed. 1998. *Functional Somatic Syndromes: Etiology, Diagnosis, and Treatment.* Cambridge, UK: Cambridge University Press.

McMahon, B.T., and L.R. Shaw. 2000. *Enabling Lives: Biographies of Six Prominent Americans with Disabilities.* Boca Raton, FL: CRC.

Melhorn, J.M., J.B. Talmage, W.E. Ackerman, and M.H. Hyman, eds. 2014. *AMA Guides to the Evaluation of Disease and Injury Causation.* Second edition. Chicago: American Medical Association.

Moynihan, R., and **A. Cassels.** 2005. *Selling Sickness: How the World's Biggest Pharmaceutical Companies Are Turning Us All Into Patients.* New York: Nations.

Neel, A.B., and **B. Hogan.** 2012. *Are Your Prescriptions Killing You? How to Prevent Dangerous Interactions, Avoid Deadly Side Effects, and Be Healthier with Fewer Drugs.* New York: Atria.

Null, G. 2009. *Death by Medicine.* Mt. Jackson, VA: Pratikos.

Organization for Economic Co-Operation and Development. 2003. *Transforming Disability Into Ability: Policies to Promote Work and Income Security for Disabled People.* Paris: Organisation for Economic Co-Operation and Development.

Petersen, M. 2008. *Our Daily Meds: How the Pharmaceutical Companies Transformed Themselves Into Slick Marketing Machines and Hooked the Nation on Prescription Drugs.* New York: Sarah Crichton.

Pope, A.M., and A.R. Tarlov, eds. 1991. *Disability in America: Toward a National Agenda for Prevention.* Washington, DC: National Academy Press.

Reeve, C. 2002. *Nothing is Impossible: Reflections on a New Life.* New York: Ballantine.

Register, C. 1987. *The Chronic Illness Experience: Embracing the Imperfect Life.* Center City, MN: Hazelden.

Reid, T.R. 2010. *The Healing of America: A Global Quest for Better, Cheaper, and Fairer Health Care.* New York: Penguin Books.

Rogers, R., ed. 1988. *Clinical Assessment of Malingering and Deception.* New York: Guilford.

Rondinelli, R.D., E. Genovese, R.T. Katz, T.M. Mayer, K. Mueller, M.I. Ranavaya, and C.R. Brigham, eds. 2008. *Guides to the Evaluation of Permanent Impairment.* Sixth edition. Chicago: American Medical Association.

Rothschild, B. 2000. *The Body Remembers: The Psychophysiology of Trauma and Trauma Treatment.* New York: W.W. Norton.

Salerno, S. 2005. *Sham: How the Self-Help Movement Made America Helpless.* New York: Three Rivers.

Sampson, W., and **L. Vaughn.** 2000. *Science Meets Alternative Medicine: What the Evidence Says About Unconventional Treatments.* Amherst, NY: Prometheus.

Sarno, J.E. 1991. *Healing Back Pain: The Mind-Body Connection*. New York: Warner Books.

Sarno, J.E. 1998. *The Mindbody Prescription: Healing the Body, Healing the Pain*. New York: Warner Books.

Sarno, J.E. 2006. *The Divided Mind: The Epidemic of Mindbody Disorders*. New York: ReganBooks.

Satel, S. 2000. *PC, M.D.: How Political Correctness is Corrupting Medicine*. New York: Basic Books.

Scaer, R.C. 2007. *The Body Bears the Burden: Trauma, Dissociation, and Disease*. New York: Routledge.

Sharpe, V.A., and A.I. Faden. 1998. *Medical Harm: Historical, Conceptual, and Ethical Dimensions of Iatrogenic Illness*. Cambridge, UK: University of Cambridge Press.

Shorter, E. 1992. *From Paralysis to Fatigue: History of Psychosomatic Illness in the Modern Era*. New York: Free Press.

Showalter, E. 1997. *Hystories: Hysterical Epidemics and Modern Media*. New York: Columbia University Press.

Singh, S., and **E. Ernst.** 2008. *Trick or Treatment: The Undeniable Facts About Alternative Medicine*. New York: W.W. Norton.

Sommers, C.H., and S. Satel. 2005. *One Nation Under Therapy: How the Helping Culture is Eroding Self-Reliance*. New York: St. Martin's Griffin.

Sparrow, M.K. 2000. *License to Steal: How Fraud Bleeds America's Health Care System*. Boulder, CO: Westview.

Strand, R.D. 2003. *Death by Prescription: The Shocking Truth Behind an Overmedicated Nation*. Nashville, TN: Thomas Nelson.

Sykes, C.J. 1992. *A Nation of Victims: The Decay of the American Character*. New York: St. Martin's.

Szasz, T.S. 1974. *The Myth of Mental Illness: Foundations of a Theory of Personal Conduct*. Revised edition. New York: Perennial Library.

Szasz, T.S. 2007. *The Medicalization of Everyday Life*. Syracuse, NY: Syracuse University Press.

Talmage, J.B, J.M. Melhorn, and **M.H. Hyman,** eds. 2011. *AMA Guides to the Evaluation of Work Ability and Return to Work*. Second edition. Chicago: American Medical Association.

Ubel, P. 2006. *You're Stronger than You Think: Tapping Into the Secrets of Emotionally Resilient People*. New York: McGraw-Hill.

Ubel, P.A. 2012. *Critical Decisions: How You and Your Doctor Can Make the Right Medical Choices Together.* New York: HarperOne.

Vujicic, N.J. 2010. *Life Without Limits: Inspiration for a Ridiculously Good Life.* New York: Doubleday Religion.

Vujicic, N. 2012. *Unstoppable: The Incredible Power of Faith in Action.* Colorado Springs, CO: Waterbook Press.

Waddell, G. 1998. *The Back Pain Revolution.* Edinburg: Churchill Livingston.

Waddell, G., and **M. Aylward.** 2009. *Models of Sickness and Disability.* London: Royal Society of Medicine Press.

Waddell, G., M. Aylward, and P. Sawney. 2002. *Back Pain, Incapacity for Work, and Social Security Benefits: An International Literature Review and Analysis.* London: Royal Society of Medicine Press.

Waddell, G., and **A.K. Burton.** 2006. *Is Work Good for Your Health and Well-being?* London: UK Stationary Office.

Warren, P.A. 2011. *Behavioral Health Disability: Innovations in Prevention and Management.* New York: Springer.

Weintraub, M.I., ed. 1995. "Malingering and Conversion Reactions." *Neurologic Clinics* 13 (2): May.

Welch, H.G. 2015. *Less Medicine, More Health: Seven Assumptions That Drive Too Much Medical Care.* Boston: Beacon.

Welch, H.G., L.M. Schwartz, and **S. Woloshin.** 2011. *Overdiagnosed: Making People Sick in the Pursuit of Health.* Boston: Beacon.

Wen, L., and **J. Kosonosky.** *When Doctors Don't Listen: How to Avoid Misdiagnoses and Unnecessary Tests.* New York: Thomas Dunne.

Wennberg, J.E. 2010. *Tracking Medicine: A Researcher's Quest to Understand Health Care.* New York: Oxford University Press.

Whitaker, R. 2002. *Mad in America: Bad Science, Bad Medicine, and the Enduring Mistreatment of the Mentally Ill.* New York: Basic Books.

Whitaker, R. 2010. *Anatomy of an Epidemic: Magic Bullets, Psychiatric Drugs, and the Astonishing Rise of Mental Illness in America.* New York: Broadway Paperbacks.

Wunderlich, G.S., D.P. Rice, and N.L. Amado, eds. 2002. *The Dynamics of Disability: Measuring and Monitoring Disability for Social Security Programs.* Washington, DC: National Academy Press.

Index